Praise for *We the Patients*

"*We the Patients* belongs to every person fatigued, frustrated, and forsaken by the maze that passes for our healthcare system."
—Lisa Fitzpatrick, MD, MPH, MPA,
Former Medicaid Chief Medical Officer

"Where Thomas Paine's *Common Sense* helped ignite the American Revolution, Matthew Zachary gives voice to a new Patient Revolution. *We the Patients* is essential reading for anyone wronged by American healthcare, exposing how the system works against patients and showing how real power can be reclaimed."
—Jeremy Abbate, Publisher, *Scientific American*

"A clarion call for how we can all work together to rig the system in order to better serve the needs of patients, not corporate interests."
—Wendell Potter, Healthcare Whistleblower, Publisher and Executive Editor of *HEALTH CARE un-Covered*

"*We the Patients* restores humanity to healthcare. Matthew blends critique with hope and reminds us what's at stake when we stop listening to patients."
—Henry S. Friedman, MD, Deputy Director of the Preston Robert Tisch Brain Tumor Center at Duke

"*We the Patients* shows why medical progress means nothing without patient accountability. Required reading for anyone shaping cancer care."

—Karen E. Knudsen, MBA, PhD, CEO,
Parker Institute for Cancer Immunotherapy,
Former CEO, American Cancer Society

"*We the Patients* brilliantly explains how American healthcare got here while giving hope to millions who have felt unseen navigating it. I could not put this book down."

—Jody Hoyos, CEO, Prevent Cancer Foundation

"Matthew lays the groundwork for the coming healthcare revolution, led by cancer survivors and the people who love and care for them, to change the system that failed them."

—Lisa C. Richardson, MD, MPH, Former Division
Director, Cancer Prevention and Control at the
Centers for Disease Control and Prevention

"*We the Patients* reframes patients not as endpoints or data sources, but as essential partners in progress. This book belongs in the hands of anyone designing the future of care."

—Jessica Federer, Former Chief Digital Officer,
Bayer AG

"*We the Patients* explains why patients feel angry and lost and shows they are not failing the system. The system is failing them."

—Barb Collura, Former CEO, RESOLVE:
The National Infertility Association

"*We the Patients* gives voice to the people who live inside the data. Matthew shows how stories and science together can make healthcare more honest and more human."
                    —Jim Weiss, Founder & Chairman, Real Chemistry

"Matthew has bent Every Which Way (and Loose) to advocate for We the Patients since he was first diagnosed with brain cancer as a 21-year-old. Now, three decades later, he's making the case for *We the Patients*, armed with data, raw stories, and a burning platform."
                    —Jane Sarasohn-Kahn, Health Economist and
                              Founder/Blogger at Health Populi

WE THE PATIENTS

WE THE PATIENTS

UNDERSTANDING, NAVIGATING, AND SURVIVING
AMERICA'S HEALTHCARE NIGHTMARE

MATTHEW ZACHARY
WITH **JEN SINGER**

WILEY

Published by John Wiley & Sons, Inc., Hoboken, New Jersey.

For general information on our other products and services or for technical support, please contact our Customer Care Department within the United States at (800) 762-2974, outside the United States at (317) 572-3993 or fax (317) 572-4002.

Wiley also publishes its books in a variety of electronic formats. Some content that appears in print may not be available in electronic formats. For more information about Wiley products, visit our website at www.wiley.com.

Library of Congress Cataloging-in-Publication Data is Available:

ISBN 9781394381333 (Cloth)
ISBN 9781394381340 (ePub)
ISBN 9781394381357 (ePDF)

Cover Design: Jon Boylan
Cover Image: © sjgh/Shutterstock
Author Photo: © B. Freed Photography
Printed and bound by CPI Group (UK) Ltd, Croydon, CR0 4YY

C9781394381333_020426

For the souls who didn't live long enough to see the system change.

For the ones still buried in paperwork instead of peace.

For the families who mortgaged their futures to buy another month.

For the parents who watered down baby food to pay for chemo.

For the advocates who keep pushing the boulder anyway.

For the nurses who stayed late, the doctors who told the truth, and the navigators who refused to hang up.

For everyone still fighting for care they never should have had to earn.

For the millions who wake up every day inside a system that treats survival like a transaction.

For the kid I was when this started—terrified, angry, and stubborn enough to live long enough to write this.

This book belongs to you.

We the patients.

Contents

Foreword

If you have ever wondered why the American healthcare system is so effective at making profits for corporations and so ineffective at making it easy for patients to get the care they need, then you've picked up the right book.

I first met Matthew Zachary at the 2012 OMG! Cancer Summit for Young Adults in Las Vegas. Gathered in a conference room at the Palms Casino, I had the opportunity to share my experiences as a former insurance industry executive turned whistleblower in front of a room full of adolescent and young adult cancer survivors and patients. Like Matthew, each person in that conference room had endured the unnecessary and burdensome pain that comes with being seriously ill in America. As if getting treatment for a cancer diagnosis wasn't enough to be dealing with, each person at that summit was all too familiar with the experience of listening to hours of hold music, trying to resolve a disputed claim with their insurance company, and in many cases, ultimately being told that what they needed would not be covered and that they would need to find a way to pay for imaging, testing, radiation, or chemotherapy out of pocket.

We gathered under the roof of a casino, where tourists willingly came to gamble despite unlikely odds. In some respects, the people gathered for that summit were also forced to gamble. In fighting cancer, they had to gamble with their lives, hoping that one treatment or another would treat their illness and result in remission. But perhaps an even bigger gamble was to have the audacity to ask their insurers to cover the cost of their care. Insurance in the American healthcare system is a gamble. Big Insurance conglomerates run the US health-care casino, and just like in Vegas, the house usually wins.

During my time in the insurance industry, I had the unfortunate duty of persuading the American public and their elected officials that the insurance industry is a necessary component of our health-care system. Simply put, I was responsible for creating propaganda that advanced the interests of greedy shareholders that own those insurance conglomerates. After many years of watching families torn apart by unnecessary grief and seeing my own neighbors seeking medical care in horse stables near where I grew up in rural Tennessee, I left the insurance industry and vowed to speak out against my former employers. This book serves to dispel the innumerable lies that corporate interests use to maintain the status quo of our health-care system.

Matthew provides a clear and concise historical retelling of the American healthcare system, sharing insights about the villains who shaped it to their financial advantage, as well as the heroes who have worked tirelessly over the past century to reform it. The book includes practical tips on how patients can turn the tables and rig the healthcare system in their favor, and Matthew makes a clarion call for how we can all work together to rig the system in order to better serve the needs of patients, not corporate interests. Matthew's journey is one of true inspiration, not because he fought and beat his cancer, nor because of his subsequent activism, though his continued advocacy is admirable. Rather, Matthew inspires me and so many others in the fight for a better healthcare system by centering the interests of patients as a core principle of future reforms. Patients are more than their diagnosis, and they are not victims of illness. As Matthew says in this book, they are individuals with agency who can and must unite in order to rig the healthcare system to increase the odds that they can live a longer and better life.

We the Patients dissects the intersection of corporate greed and political inaction in our healthcare system. From the excessive use of prior authorization to the narrowing of provider networks, corporations have continued to invent new and terrible ways to squeeze profit out of our healthcare system. Legislative efforts over the past half century have entirely failed to adequately protect patients and consumers.

If you are someone who is sick and tired of a healthcare system that is not designed to serve your interests, this book will give you the practical steps you need to join the growing movement of health-care consumers who are ready for things to change.

—*Wendell Potter*
Editor and Publisher, *HEALTH CARE un-covered*
Philadelphia, PA

Preface

I'm twenty-one years old, and my father is driving me home from treatments for brain cancer when he comes upon a disabled truck blocking Manhattan's 51st Street. We're stuck. Cars begin lining up behind us, and several are honking, because, New York. The driver of the truck shrugs like an Italian soccer player after a foul and turns his back on us all. My father sighs—and then drives up onto the curb, across the sidewalk, and back onto the street on the other side of the broken truck just to get me back home.

If that's not a metaphor for the ways that patients have to navigate the fuckery that is the American healthcare system, I don't know what is. The roadblocks from insurance companies. The anger of the patients and their families. The indifference of the system. The on-the-spot workarounds that may not work next time. It's all in the way of accessing healthcare. Only, in the case of America's healthcare system, it's not broken; it was *designed* that way.

After thirty years into my remission and a lifetime as, says *People* magazine, "the people's voice in healthcare," I've discovered the trick to surviving our convoluted healthcare system: *Don't try to fix it. Rig it in your favor.*

Ever since Kaiser Permanente persuaded President Nixon to privatize American health insurance in 1973, the system has been working exactly the way it was designed: to put patients at the bottom of the funnel for maximum profits at the top. Your chemotherapy, radiation treatments, immunotherapy, surgery, tests, medications, and care cost them money, cutting into their profits. So, they put up roadblocks like prior authorizations and claim delays and denials to improve their bottom line, often at your expense.

For the tens of millions of Americans who each year face illness, both acute and chronic, it's a prescription to be pissed. And if the public's near-gleeful reaction to the murder of a health insurance company CEO is any indication,[i] patients have had it with the American healthcare system. It's hard enough to navigate your own diagnosis, the treatments, their side effects, and your now upside-down life, but it's doubly difficult when your care and your outcome are predicated on the answer to a single question: "What insurance do you have?"

In *We the Patients: Understanding, Navigating, and Surviving America's Healthcare Nightmare,* I'll investigate how we got into this mess in the first place, mired by a system that's geared more toward profits than patients. Then I'll offer up a fresh solution for the healthcare, um, malignant malfeasance (my mom says I'm using too many f-words) that gets in our way of affordable, quality care—and if the pandemic taught us anything, it's that no one gets a healthcare hall pass. I'll start an IV drip of knowing compassion and wisdom from my wide network of patient advocates and policy wonks. They'll do rounds with us to help you get unscrewed by the system, review the history behind the patient rights you probably didn't even know you had, and navigate you—and all of us—across the harsh seas of the system. It's not about fixing the complicated for-profit system so much as it's about protecting patients from the worst of it.

Just like chemo, *We the Patients* will make you feel worse before you feel better, diagnosing America's healthcare nightmare before showing you how to channel anger into a new kind of advocacy that's being crafted for these tenuous times. I'll share how I got my (new) life back after a life-threatening, golf ball-sized, rare brain tumor ended my piano career. Turns out, I was born with cancer.

---

[i] For the record: murder = bad.

Luckily, I was also born with congenital chutzpah. I went from "You're going to die" to survivor to nationally recognized cancer rebel, patient advocate, community builder, podcast hero, and unapologetic healthcare disrupter.

Making healthcare suck less has long been my crusade, first as the founder of the award-winning nonprofit organization Stupid Cancer, the largest adolescent and young adult (AYA) cancer community in the world. There, I served as a midwife to the young adult cancer movement, shining a light on a demographic long neglected in cancer care. Together, we tackled the isolation often experienced by patients who don't fit neatly into pediatric or older adult patient groups. We met in person at CancerCon, our annual event for AYAs to commiserate, kvetch, and keep an eye on one another, patient to patient, survivor to survivor.

We talked about our diagnoses and our treatments, the side effects, the stares from people in supermarkets and restaurants trying to decide if we'd shaved our heads for a mosh pit or for a terrible diagnosis that we were "too young for." We also talked about something uniquely American: a crumbling healthcare system that's driven by profit margins.

Now it's time to put all that I've learned from my diverse and brilliant network, who have shopped at the Shit Happens Store that is healthcare, to provide a solution—a patient protections movement that I could have used back when my dad forged a new path in front of the corner pharmacy.

We the Patients is a proclamation for our times, when two-thirds of all bankruptcies[1] are medical, medicine is political, and inequities are baked into the healthcare pie. It's a raw, entertaining, and informative exploration of what happens when healthcare goes wrong and how to make it right.

There are now an estimated 19 million cancer survivors, and nowadays, about half of cancers are diagnosed at lower stages, increasing the odds of survivorship.[2] By 2040, our numbers are expected to hit 26 million.[3] Together with our families, we make up a sizable and formidable voting bloc. We can learn how to rig the system that is healthcare by changing it from the inside out.

It's time for a unifying, nonpartisan political movement with trusted leadership to lead the next great sea change in patient protections. It's about time for a healthcare system where every patient has timely, affordable, and comprehensive care—one that respects the human cost of illness and eliminates the systemic barriers that prevent better outcomes while allowing the for-profit healthcare system to remain for-profit.

It's time for *We the Patients*, the book, and We the Patients, the movement. Together, nothing can get in our way.

PROCLAMATION
WE THE PATIENTS . . .
We have had enough.
We have a moral reckoning.
We have a national reckoning.

No more prior authorizations.
No more robot denials.
No more appeals.

We are not out of network.
We are stronger than any insurance claim.
We are louder than any denial letter.

We are for every patient who ever died waiting for prior authorization and claim approvals.
We are for every family that went broke just trying to live.
We are for every loved one lost to a denied claim.
We are not here to raise awareness.
We are not waiting for permission.
We are not to be placed on hold.

We have the right to a healthcare system designed to help, not harm.
We the survivors.
We the caregivers.
We the parents.
We the veterans.
We the grieving.
We the people.

WE THE PATIENTS.

1

We the Nightmare

The American healthcare system was crafted, designed, and calibrated to operate exactly as it does: squeezing profits at the expense of real care. To find out why, we need to travel back in time to the seventies and listen in on a conversation between President Nixon and his aide John Ehrlichman, who was explaining the thinking behind what would become the Health Maintenance Organization (HMO) Act of 1973 as an "alternative to existing fee-for-service medical care."[1] Ehrlichman had reportedly spoken with Edgar Kaiser, Jr., who ran his father's company, Kaiser Permanente, among the largest healthcare conglomerates then and now.

Ehrlichman told Nixon, "Edgar Kaiser is running his Permanente deal for profit. And the reason that he can . . . the reason he can do it . . . All the incentives are toward less medical care, because the less care they give them, the more money they make."[2]

It's not that it was illegal to profit from US healthcare before the act was passed. It's that the 1973 act exempted HMOs from state laws that limited medical decisions to doctors. And that had a direct effect on why your insurance company—and not your doctor—has the final say in whether you're getting that PET scan your oncologist ordered to check whether you're in remission. As PolitiFact put it decades later, "As a result, the medical practice was subject to more corporate influence."[3] The HMO Act opened up alternatives to the existing healthcare system, and soon, HMOs began to proliferate.[4]

I was born one year after the HMO Act was passed, but I like to imagine healthcare before it to be like the TV show *Marcus Welby, MD*, about a primary care doctor who made house calls in a blue suit and a dab of Brylcreem, advising everyone from pregnant hippies to asthmatic priests about their health and their lives. Back then, doctors had ample time to spend with their patients, the autonomy to make diagnoses and treatment plans without interference from insurance companies, and a billing process void of middlemen.

Since then, the relationship between private interests (read: massive profit) and public health, coupled with the institutional inequities that prevails, has spawned nearly every egregious healthcare injustice on American soil. Every argument you've had with insurance companies, every delay in care while you waited for a prior authorization, every alarming Explanation of Benefits equal to the price of a used Toyota Corolla, every time you worried about losing your health insurance along with your job, can be traced back to this massive shift toward massive profit.

We all have to shop for healthcare, yet it isn't exactly retail. No one asks to get sick, which means that the healthcare sector is a supply-driven or a supply-influenced economy. There's no demand to get chemotherapy until you need it, and no one matriculates at Cancer University to learn how to navigate treatments. Compare that with shopping for a new fridge or a car in a sector where there's lots of demand and endless reviews to help you figure out what to buy.

Meanwhile, doctors and many other medical professionals are also screwed by Big Insurance, which is why visiting your GP often feels like being on a 15-minute in/out assembly line. Doctors are so frustrated, in fact, that an increasing number are opting out of the system entirely to become "concierge doctors" or to practice "membership medicine," further widening the economic gap between those who can afford good healthcare and those who have to scrape together whatever they can get. Some have taken to social media to "out" health insurance companies that, they say, impinged on their ability to practice medicine through delays and denials. Meanwhile, pharmacists are burnt out and pharmacies are under-staffed, and the nursing shortage is expected to come up about 63,000 RNs short by 2030.[5]

In other words, everyone is getting screwed except . . . shareholders? CEOs?

Yeah, I went there. Look at how a vocal group of people reacted to the murder of UnitedHealthcare CEO Brian Thompson, which happened on a Manhattan sidewalk in late 2024. Nearly 30,000 people would soon contribute to the legal defense for Thompson's alleged murderer Luigi Mangione—the antihero I didn't have on my healthcare bingo card—raising more than a million bucks.[6] Soon, #FreeLuigi became a social media go-to for this unusual fan club. Let me be clear: I'm not an advocate of murder. The fact that I even have to write that shows just how pissed off Americans are about the current state of health insurance. They understand that it's not so much about the patients as it is about the profits.

Here's a sliver of a reason why they're so pissed: UnitedHealth Group was making incredible amounts of money. Billions. In fact, their 2024 revenues grew $28.7 billion, or 8 percent year over year, to $400.3 billion, ranking at the top of the industry.[7] But after their CEO was murdered, the market forced them to adjust the way they did business, at least temporarily, and some of their investors weren't happy about it.

In early 2025, investors filed a class action suit against UnitedHealthcare for "failure to disclose the shift away from its previously aggressive claim denial strategies and the resulting impact on profitability."[8] Their chief complaint? The company had promised them mo' money, but then it slashed its projected earnings. As Reuters reported, UnitedHealthcare was sued for "allegedly concealing how backlash from the killing of a top executive was damaging its business, causing its stock to nosedive after the insurer lowered its 2025 outlook." After the filing, says Benzinga, "UnitedHealthcare stock plunged 22.4 percent, wiping out approximately $119 billion in market value in one day."[9]

These investors were unabashedly and publicly pissed off that the company seemed to have cut back on its "deny, delay, defend" methods of insurance (dis)approvals. The same process, increasingly fueled by artificial intelligence, had caused the company's denial rates through Medicare Advantage to surge from 10.9 percent in 2020 to 22.7 percent in 2022, a U.S. Senate investigation reported.[10]

Before the murder, UnitedHealthcare was stamping a big fat "NO" on more and more insurance claims. Need an "investigational" surgery or immunotherapy? A robot says it's "not medically necessary," so, no. After the murder, they quietly pulled back on their process of rejection and the market spoke.

Didn't We Almost Have It All?

The global pandemic taught us that no one gets a healthcare hall pass except Big Insurance, which made record profits during the ordeal and, while no one was paying attention, eroded consumer rights.

Unlike nearly every other place on Earth, healthcare in America is personal *and* political, with an unconscionably heaping dose of institutional inequality baked in. If you're socioeconomically disadvantaged, come from a marginalized community, or were just born in the wrong zip code, you're doubly screwed. And since two-thirds of all bankruptcies are medical,[11] it's likely you or someone you know has been triply screwed by crushing medical debt.

Decades before the HMO Act of 1973 unleashed the havoc that led us to where our healthcare system is today, we had a shot at universal healthcare—and we missed the basket with a thud. In the early twentieth century, many European countries adopted nationalized healthcare, but not us. Beginning in 1883 clear through to 1912, countries including Austria, Britain, Denmark, Germany, Hungary, Norway, Russia, Sweden, and Switzerland adopted some form of "compulsory sickness insurance" to protect workers from economic ruin due to illness. It was the precursor to universal healthcare guaranteeing coverage to all citizens that Europeans seem to take for granted, like their outdoor cafés, efficient train travel, and bread with just three ingredients.

What was America doing while all this healthcare reform was going on overseas? They left it to the states, because 'Murica. Though President Theodore Roosevelt supported health insurance for workers, much of the efforts for reform at the time happened at the local and state level. Then in 1915, a committee on social welfare introduced a bill to provide healthcare for the least fortunate of the working class, offering coverage up to a certain income level. The early plans called for a split in financial responsibility to cover medical aid and sick pay: 40 percent by workers, 40 percent by employers, and 20 percent by the state.[12]

The American Medical Association (AMA) supported it, but the American Federation of Labor denounced it, claiming it would create a paternalistic control over Americans' health. It would also screw with the unions' collective bargaining. Private insurance, meanwhile, opposed the bill largely because it would provide coverage for funeral expenses, which was their jam, and the life insurance industry stood to lose millions of dollars.[13]

Then there was hatred for all things German that arose during World War I, and Germany had been the first country to offer what opponents in America called "socialist insurance." In certain circles, it was considered un-American, if not downright communist, to provide citizens with health insurance, a sentiment that would stand the test of time well into the twenty-first century. But this was the era of the Red Scare, when Americans feared communist influence in our country, and state-backed healthcare was considered a dangerous example of the "Prussian menace" that some felt threatened America's freedom.

Then in the 1920s, there was a shift from efforts to protect workers from being devastated by sickness to being decimated by healthcare costs as medical innovations came to market. Among the medical inventions of the Roaring Twenties were insulin, the EEG to measure brain activity, the Pap smear, and the iron lung, and these things cost money. Hospitals began to shift from the place you went to die to the place you went for a cure. Soon, Americans' concerns shifted, too, from fears of illness stealing their earning power to medical costs wiping out their bank accounts. Doctors started charging more to cover licensing fees and also simply because they could, and by 1929, hospital costs made up about 13 percent of the average family's medical bills.[14] It was getting expensive to get well.

So a bunch of frustrated AMA members—all muckety-mucks from the likes of Johns Hopkins, the Brookings Institution, Yale, and the Boston Medical Dispensary (no, not *that* kind of dispensary)— got together to form the Committee on the Costs of Medical Care (CCMC). They were funded by major private foundations with names like Rockefeller. By the time the CCMC issued their main report on the state of American healthcare in 1932, they had 48 members, including physicians, public health officials, economists, and hospital administrators.

Their recommendations, issued in a report called "Medical Care for the American People" in the earliest years of the Great Depression, included:

1. Comprehensive medical care provided by practitioners and hospitals
2. Basic public health services for the entire population
3. Medical costs paid by groups through insurance, taxation, or both, or individual fee-for-service
4. Urban and rural coordination through the formation of state and local agencies
5. Improved professional education for healthcare providers[15]

But certain people went batshit crazy about the report. The AMA called it an "incitement to revolution."[16] *The New York Times* used the "S" word, calling it "socialized medicine" in a front-page headline,[17] and other newspapers pretty much echoed the sentiment. Even Dr. William J. Mayo, co-founder of the esteemed Mayo Clinic which was already using a system like the one proposed, backed the AMA's stance against it.[18]

This is why we can't have nice things.

The report, which was co-signed by 35 of the 48 members of the CCMC, said the plan would "provide for the first time a scientific basis on which communities throughout the country can attack the perplexing problem of providing adequate medical care for all persons, at costs within their means" through subsidized fees. But a bunch of doctors were having none of it.

Why? Deep in the bowels of the website for the nonprofit foundation Milbank Memorial Fund, a paper from 1933 sums up the report and the response to it. Swap out the numbers and it could easily have been written about today's healthcare system:

> Sickness falls alike on the rich and the poor, the survey reveals, and yet nearly two million families in the United States, whose incomes are less than $1,200 a year, 'receive no professional medical or dental attention of any kind, curative or preventive,' and this 'in spite of the large volume of free work done by hospitals, health departments, and individual practitioners, and in spite of the sliding scale of charges.' However, even the well-to-do families receive less medical care than they should have, according to standards accepted by the Committee. Most Americans stay away from dentists . . . Preventive medicine is still little used.[19]

Yet the *Journal of the American Medical Association* (*JAMA*), still today a prestigious medical journal, said in 1932 that the plan would mean the destruction of private practice and that the recommendations in the CCMC's report "represent exploitation of physicians for the gain of business."[20] The editors called the involvement of government in healthcare an "invasion" and a "curse."

A few members of the CCMC also issued a Minority Report, and I don't mean the Tom Cruise movie, and it was more popular than the "socialist manifesto" that the dissenters perceived the Majority Report to be. Mostly, it railed against the costs associated with the report's recommendations, but it also took issue with the idea of medicine provided by groups instead of individual practices. The signers of the chief Minority Report (the second, by two dentists, wasn't as popular) said they were "not opposed to insurance but only to the abuses and evils that have practically always accompanied insurance medicine."[21]

The effects of the chief Minority Report can still be felt today because, you may have noticed, we still don't have universal healthcare, yet we do have Medicare and Medicaid.[i] Launched in the 1960s, these programs have their roots in the CCMC's Majority Report. The Minority Report, on the other hand, helped lead us to minimal government intervention, and it's why every time a "pro-business" politician, a C-suite insurance executive, or a Facebook troll calls universal healthcare "socialized medicine," a healthcare insurance lobbyist gets their wings.

President Franklin Delano Roosevelt could have guaranteed us healthcare, but he chose not to put it into the Social Security Act in 1935, fearing that the AMA—a very strong lobby at the time— would sink the whole thing.[22] Some say he made up his mind during a lunch with a neurosurgeon relative the day before introducing the Act. So the next time you need a prior auth, thank FDR? Oh, but there are so many more people to thank . . . .[23]

It's Not Dead Yet

The quest for universal healthcare didn't die with the Depression. Beginning in 1943, three Congressmen tried to get us national health insurance by introducing and re-introducing a bill in various forms every year for fourteen years. Senator Robert F. Wagner of New York,

---

[i] As of this writing, Medicaid still exists.

Senator James E. Murray of Montana, and John Dingell, Sr.[ii] of Michigan proposed and kept on proposing the Wagner-Murray-Dingell bill in an attempt to establish a national health insurance program funded by payroll taxes, like Social Security.

They defended the bill in the 1945 Congressional Record, with Wagner writing, "Prepaid medical care is not socialized medicine," adding that these are "devil words" created by propagandists to confuse the issue: "A system of prepaid medical care is simply a method of assuring a person ready access to the medical care that he or she needs by eliminating the financial barrier between the patient and doctor or hospital."[24]

It sounds so simple and sensible when you take out the devil words, doesn't it? But of course, it failed over and over again. Along the way, President Harry S. Truman introduced an even more ambitious plan that would make its way into the trio's bill, proposing that a federal healthcare system would be funded through payroll taxes, in 1945. This time, the funeral payment plan that had torpedoed earlier efforts was dropped to make the insurance companies happy.

Still, it didn't pass because of the usual congressional bullshit. Led by an anti-union conservative, the House committee in charge of health insurance refused to even hold hearings.[25] Then Senator Robert A. Taft of Ohio called it, "the most socialistic measure this Congress has ever had before it,"[26] though he believed in government-sponsored healthcare coverage for the poor. The AMA fought against what they saw as a loss of doctors' autonomy to the government.[27] The AMA even launched a PR campaign to combat support for universal healthcare, featuring some ~~propaganda~~ cartoons that, in another era, would have been shared widely on fringe social media feeds (Figure 1.1).

Then the soldiers came home.

[ii] If you're thinking, *Wait a minute. I remember Dingell.* That was likely his son, John Dingell, Jr., who holds the record for longest time in office: nearly 60 years.

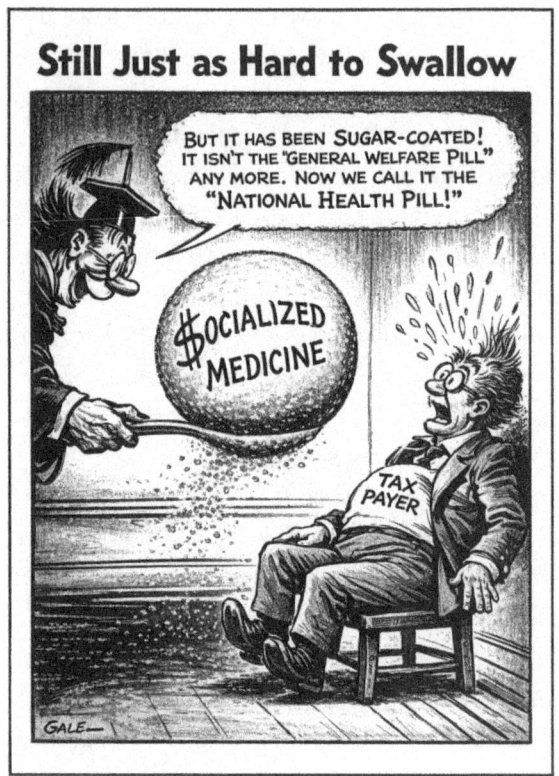

FIGURE 1.1   Still Just as Hard to Swallow.
Source: New York Journal-American, mid-20th century

To thwart inflation in the post-war boom, the US government imposed caps on wages. To lure workers during the growing economy, companies began to offer employer-sponsored health insurance, and the IRS later sealed the deal by declaring employer contributions to health insurance tax exempt.[28] See? They call them benefits, but they aren't just good for the employee . . . who may now be trapped in a soul-sucking, dead-end job because they need the insurance. Healthcare in America was now officially tied to work.

In the 1950s, President Dwight D. Eisenhower sought to bring down the costs of health insurance by enrolling more people in employer-sponsored plans. More healthy enrollees means more money for sick ones. While just 6 percent of the population had health insurance in 1939, by the end of the 1950s, nearly 70 percent did.[29] Who do you think didn't? Employment benefits in the 1950s were mostly for the benefit of men. Think: *The Man in the Gray Flannel Suit*, Don Draper look-alikes working in office buildings, or Ralph Kramden-types with union jobs down at the factory or in public utilities. If you weren't a white man or married to one, it was harder to get health insurance. In 1957, some three-quarters of white people had health insurance compared to just over half of Black people.[30]

The new rules provided healthcare for millions while also creating disparities. If you worked part-time or in a small business that couldn't afford healthcare, you were shit out of luck. Retirees, widows, and (mainly Hispanic) people who worked in industries like agriculture without health benefits or unions didn't have access to affordable healthcare.

It solidified the American healthcare system as a patchwork tied to employment. Or as David Blumenthal, M.D., M.P.P. wrote in the *New England Journal of Medicine* *(NEJM)* two decades ago, "The future welfare of physicians and their patients now depends vitally on an apparent accident of history that emerged seventy years ago from the throes of depression and war."[31]

Yet politicians kept on trying to make the most of the accident.

Welcome to the Jungle

In the 1960s, President Lyndon B. Johnson did what FDR wouldn't or couldn't: He guaranteed healthcare to certain marginalized groups. He signed the Social Security Amendments of 1965, allotting taxes to pay for Medicare, which provides health insurance to the elderly, and Medicaid for the poor and disabled.

How did he pull that off?

First of all, healthcare for the elderly was a popular idea in the 1960s. LBJ had help from House Ways and Means Committee chairman Wilbur Mills, a Democrat who understood what it took to get a bill providing healthcare for everyone over age sixty-five passed, including certain concessions to the AMA and the Republicans.[32] The bill made private insurers happy by taking on the "bad risk" of the growing population of old people, who tend to get sick more often than other demographics.[33] Plus, the bill was framed not as a new-fangled, scary thing, but as a logical extension of Social Security.

Some of the usual suspects shouted, "Socialism!" But most people supported the idea of making sure that the care for Grandpa's heart attack was covered by insurance. Medicare and Social Security ultimately helped turn the elderly into a powerful voting bloc that tends to turn out in elections. In 2024, for instance, more than 70 percent of Americans 65 and older voted, while a little more than half of 25 to 44-year-olds did.[34]

Back in the sixties, Medicare cost $10 billion a year to fund. By the 2020s, however, that cost had ballooned to $830 billion, accounting for 20 percent of the healthcare spending in the United States.[35] Over the decades since its inception, Medicare has undergone its share of changes, including an expansion to cover people with disabilities, in 1972, and in 2003, the addition of prescription drug coverage, that "Medicare Part D" you hear about on commercials during "The Golden Girls" reruns on waiting room TVs.

In the 1990s, President Bill Clinton once again attempted to introduce universal health coverage for all Americans, putting his wife, First Lady Hillary Clinton, in charge, and so, people began calling it "Hillarycare." But the Health Insurance Association of America spent about $20 million on an opposition advertising campaign known as the "Harry and Louise" commercials. They starred a middle-aged white couple sitting at the kitchen table, surrounded by bills, yellow legal pads, and a calculator, lamenting about government-sponsored healthcare: "Having choices we don't like is no choice at all."[36]

The Clintons' plan died on the vine, but it paved its way for the Big Daddy, 2010's Affordable Care Act (ACA). You might know it as "Obamacare." Not only did it expand healthcare coverage to include preventive care, like mammograms for people on Medicare, it also expanded Medicaid coverage for low-income individuals, prevented insurers from denying coverage based on health history (ahem, cancer survivors), and established health insurance marketplaces where all sorts of people could find and buy government-subsidized insurance plans.

Got a chronic cancer that requires long-term medications? Just got a positive pregnancy test? Fighting depression? Thanks to the ACA, not only can't you be denied coverage for your "pre-existing condition," you can't be charged more, either. For now. In the first seven years of the ACA, Republicans tried to repeal, defund, or alter it some seventy times[37] (see Chapter 2), and they managed to repeal the individual mandate that required everyone to buy health insurance—that "healthy ones providing more money for sick ones" that Eisenhower had managed to push through for private plans.

In his first term, President Donald Trump promised to replace Obamacare with "something terrific," but whatever it was, it failed to materialize.[38] Then in his second term, he proposed and passed the "One Big Beautiful Bill" (OBBB), which included cuts that would likely leave millions without medical insurance at all.[39] Under the guise of cutting waste and fraud, the bill required the Energy and Commerce Committee to cut $880 billion from their budget. Which of their line items costs about $880 billion a year? You guessed it, Medicaid.[40]

The bill passed and, as of this writing, it's expected to cut millions off from Medicaid coverage over the coming decade, wreak havoc in the ACA marketplace, raise rates for the uninsured, close rural hospitals and clinics, and negatively affect nursing homes.[41]

Now we really can't have nice things. Nice, live-saving things.

The Greatest Shitshow on Earth

President after president has tried to fix the mess that is the American healthcare system, except for one in particular who has taken a chainsaw to it. To me, it's all just more clowns in the car, but it's the same car—a tiny Fiat, driving in circles around the town square. More and more clowns squeeze in, and yet, that little Fiat keeps running. Only, these days, patients are running behind the car.

Take, for example, GLP-1 drugs that lots of people are taking for weight loss. You'd think that if a doctor prescribes you a drug, you just go to your pharmacy and pick it up, right? Hahahaha, JK, you know that's not where this story is going.

In 2025, CVS Caremark, a pharmacy benefit management (PBM) division of CVS Health, decided to stop carrying the GLP-1 Zepbound in favor of another, cheaper one, called Wegovy, effectively sending the Fiat in circles for millions of patients nationwide who get their GLP-1 meds from CVS.[42]

Let's unpack what all that means in English. PBMs act as middlemen between insurance providers, pharmaceutical companies, and pharmacies (see Chapter 2). They negotiate drug prices and choose formularies, which are lists of medications that are covered and carried by pharmacies. Caremark decided to replace Zepbound with Wegovy on its formulary, so that if you tried to fill a prescription for Zepbound at one of CVS's 9,000 pharmacies, you would go home empty-handed.

No biggie, right? Just take Wegovy instead. But it absolutely can be a biggie when the medication your doctor prescribed gets substituted by someone who is not your doctor. Let's say you've been on Zepbound for months and it's worked. You've lost weight, your blood sugar levels are lower, and so is your blood pressure. You tolerate it well and you're happy and so is your doctor.

Then a PBM declares, "Now you get *this* drug instead." You might have side effects and it might not work as well. In fact, a study in the *NEJM* found Wegovy not to be as effective as Zepbound.[43] But Caremark had negotiated a deal with Novo Nordisk, the makers of Wegovy, and in these kinds of deals, *The New York Times* reported, "manufacturers also pay fees to PBMs. Those fees can add up to hundreds of millions of dollars for the biggest blockbusters."[44] These $500-a-month GLP-1s are the blockbusters of the 2020s.

Now imagine that the drug in question is your chemo, or the one anti-nausea med you've found to work, or a blood thinner that, unlike its competitor, has successfully thwarted blood clots, because that's an actual thing that happened when Caremark took Eliquis off its formulary. (It was reinstated six months later.)[45]

It's all just another clown in the car. Who gets affected? We the patients, leaving us to figure yet another workaround.

We the Fed Up

For thirty years, I've been finding workarounds for the system. I was a 21-year-old college student when I had brain cancer, so I was on my dad's health insurance, a tier one union-sponsored plan, during treatments. Even though my dad's plan was the gold standard for teacher's union health insurance in New York City, it didn't cover Memorial Sloan Kettering Cancer Center, where I had my radiation treatments. So Dad took out a catastrophe policy with a separate nightmare of a company that made his life a miserable hell for years, making him fight for every prior authorization and every claim. Dad said, "I had paperwork that made paperwork."

Our insurance would cover just $285 of my $1,650 treatments. That's *each*, and I had thirty-three of them. That math works out to about forty-five grand, and in all, my family spent $50,000 out of pocket, about $100,000 in today's money. It's not like my parents were loaded. They were schoolteachers, and Dad had all sorts of side hustles: silversmithing, student mentoring, teaching night school. He tapped into the equity in his house to cover the insane bills coming in, rationalizing, "Hey, it's only a refi." I don't know how many times my parents mortgaged the house to keep me alive. But my dad said, "When it comes to health, there is no budget."

Then I went into remission, graduated from college, and got kicked off Dad's insurance at 22 back before Obamacare covered offspring up to age 26. I needed insurance to cover my post-treatment healthcare, including the 17 prescription medications I took every day and multiple MRIs, but I didn't have a job until that fall.

So I went on COBRA. That's an acronym for the Consolidated Omnibus Budget Reconciliation Act, which was passed during the Reagan era to ensure that workers and their families could continue their employer-sponsored health insurance for up to three years after losing their job, or in my case, aging out as a son on my dad's plan. Only, it costs a small fortune. In 1997, I paid about $3,200 a year for COBRA, the equivalent of about $6,600 today.

When I finally got a job in advertising, the agency's insurance plan didn't cover my oncologist or the MRI scans to keep an eye out for any tumors returning to my brain. So I kept on paying for COBRA. To afford it, I moonlighted as a computer tech back before Geek Squad was a thing.

If this had happened after 2010, I might have been able to find a cheaper government-subsidized plan through the ACA that covered my doctors. Or not. "If you like your doctor, you will be able to keep your doctor" turned out to be an empty promise, just another clown in the car.

In America, no healthcare "journey" is taken without outsized influence by the health insurance plan you happen to have at diagnosis. It was and still is a big part of every patient's story, influencing your experience and your outcome. But it shouldn't be. Yet it would affect every patient I interviewed, every member of our organization.

As I write this, Aetna announced that it's pulling out of the ACA marketplace in 2026, leaving about a million people without healthcare coverage in 17 states. This, reports *Health Care un-covered*, right as the company enjoyed nearly $2 billion in quarterly profits.[46] That's *quarterly* with a Q. Three months. But they say they can't make enough money off Obamacare, so they're ditching it and all the patients along with it.

This isn't about Aetna or any one company or politician. It's about the constant and consistent growth of healthcare nonsense that patients have to navigate. Like my father driving up on the sidewalk to get me home, patients are met with roadblocks left and right. And somewhere along the way, somebody replaced Dad's Chevy Blazer with an overloaded Fiat—and that thing doesn't navigate the curbs as well.

No wonder the patients are so pissed. We live in a country where healthcare is not a right. Rather, it's a hodgepodge of employer-sponsored and Obamacare insurance, ever-changing laws, political power plays, and profit motive competing with patients' number one goal: to get healthy and stay alive. It's time we find the permanent workaround so that We the Patients don't have to endure any health-care . . . malevolent chicanery (better, Mom?) anymore.

Here's what I know: The revolution will, in fact, be televised. Only, probably on YouTube. Stay tuned and join us because we know a better way there.

2

We the Delayed and Denied

America suffers from a Sisyphusian buffet of healthcare nonsense, where patient advocates work hard to solve a problem only to have the powers-that-be create a new one. We fix something, and they find a way around it. We create a protection, and they locate a loophole. They do anything and everything they can to continue to make money, no matter how much it screws us over.

Though we've come a long way from the days when healthcare could reject us for the audacity of having a pre-existing condition,[i] back when you could get fired from your job for a cancer diagnosis, it's been quite the hurdle race to get here.

First, we demanded to be treated like humans instead of being left to die.

We jumped that hurdle.

Then we asked to have agency during our treatments, to be recognized as more than our disease.

---

[i]Thanks to a 2017 executive order, there's still a way: short-term insurance plans are exempt from denying coverage for pre-existing conditions. States can choose to allow, regulate, or ban them, proving that when it comes to your health, real estate agents are spot on: "Location, location, location."

We cleared that hurdle.

Then we said, "Hey, you know we're surviving more now but that's messed with our well-being. Little help here?"

We made it over that hurdle, too.

We dared to say the word *cancer* out loud, and we baked protections for pre-existing conditions into nearly all of our healthcare coverage. (Thanks, Obama.) We secured long-term survivorship support and demanded patient navigation. We asked for help transitioning from pediatric to adult cancer care, and we worked to close the gap in care for marginalized communities.

We made it through a sixty-year obstacle course, but there's still a long way to go, because they keep putting up hurdles. Often, expensive ones. Healthcare in America now costs a lot more—$14,570 per person in 2023,[1] compared to $4,884 in 2000.[2] That's more than any developed country (Figure 2.1).

The price of healthcare premiums and deductibles is just one of the many healthcare hurdles still ahead of us along this track. Even my kids' favorite cartoon, *Teen Titans Go!* spoofed the "kajillion-dollar limit" for deductibles.

"You're trying to slither your way out of covering our bill," says one of the characters to the insurance company, represented by a snake. The teens demand they cover the total cost of their hospital bill.

"Um, let me quote paragraph seven, section 6B when I say, 'Make me!'"

The teens wind up beating themselves up to incur enough costs to pay down their deductible.[3] It's a cartoonish way to show how much gets in the way of your healthcare, like for instance, God forbid, you try to use your coverage. That's when the real fuckery begins.

Delay, Deny, Defend

Diagnosed at thirty-three with a pre-cancerous condition that could have led to preventive mastectomy, Sally Neely Nix was familiar with the ways that the healthcare system can make getting healthy harder.

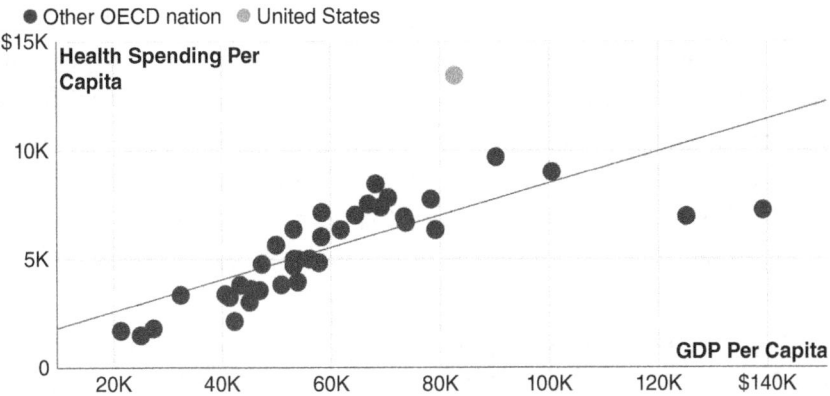

FIGURE 2.1 GDP Per Capita and Health Consumption Spending Per Capita 2023. Notes: Health spending per capita is estimated for Australia, Belgium, Costa Rica, Finland, Greece, Israel, Japan, Latvia, Mexico, the Netherlands, New Zealand, Norway, Slovak Republic, Spain, Switzerland, Türkiye, and the United States. For all other countries health spending per capita is provisional. GDP data are estimated for Colombia, Costa Rica, New Zealand, and Portugal; data are provisional for Belgium, France, Germany, Greece, Hungary, Korea, Mexico, the Netherlands, Spain, and Switzerland. Health consumption does not include investments in structures, equipment, or research.

Source: KFF analysis of OECD data. "How does health spending in the U.S. compare to other countries?" Peterson-KFF Health System Tracker, April 9, 2025. Available at https://www.healthsystemtracker.org/chart-collection/health-spending-u-s-compare-countries/

But she never expected to have to fight with her own healthcare insurance company, almost daily, to get the care prescribed by her own doctor for a painful and complex condition diagnosed in her forties. And she certainly never predicted that it would make a patient advocate out of her.

In 2011, she woke up very sick one day.

"Light hurt, sound hurt, everything hurt," she told me. Among her diagnoses were meningitis, multiple sclerosis, and trigeminal neuralgia, a condition that causes a pain so intense, it's commonly called the "suicide disease."[4] When several brain and spinal surgeries didn't bring relief, her doctor prescribed intravenous immunoglobulin infusions (IVIG). She told *KFF Health News*, "IVIG turns out to be my great hope."[5] Until it wasn't, thanks to her husband's health insurance company.

Imagine having horrific pain, finding the thing that makes you feel better, and then getting a letter from your insurance company explaining that they wouldn't cover the $13,000-a-month treatment that gave you your life back. Worse, the denial was *retroactive*, meaning she'd be stuck with the bill for the previous six months of treatments.

"They picked on the wrong person," Nix told me, and she wasn't kidding. This otherwise congenial Gen Xer with a southern drawl and a blond bob decided to fight.

"I started realizing there was no rhyme or reason to their denial." She began making phone calls. That's when she discovered that her insurance company had advised the hospital that it didn't need prior authorization, when patients and their doctors must get the okay from their insurance companies for prescriptions, treatments, or procedures.

She worked with the hospital to get documentation, including the name and phone extension of the person at her insurance company who'd assured them that no prior auth had been necessary. She discovered that her IVIG prescription was considered "investigative" while another brand was approved for use, so it wasn't covered. The difference between the two? Maybe the name? Nix said the treatments were clinically very similar but only one was covered.

She fought and won—temporarily. After receiving notice that her balance was marked paid, she restarted treatment and then— you guessed it—her insurance company found another loophole. This time it was that her diagnosis didn't qualify her for infusions.

Nix was quick to nix that, calling them out on social media and securing more than 22,000 signatures on a Change.org campaign titled, "Don't Let Profit Deny Patients Their Right to Healthcare."[6] She filed complaints with the US Department of Health and Human Services, her state's Department of Insurance and attorney general, and the US Department of Labor.

That last complaint was the charm, because the USDOL went to bat for her, asserting that her ERISA[7] rights were being violated. ERISA stands for the Employee Retirement Income Security Act of 1974, a federal law that sets minimum standards for health plans, among others. Under ERISA, private health plans must be transparent about coverage.

Nix meanwhile took to LinkedIn to call out the health insurance peer review process, where a physician, hired by your insurance company, reviews your doctor's treatment plan to determine if it's "medically necessary." Those "peers" may or may not have experience or expertise in your disease:

An OB/Gyn paid by my insurer was the so-called peer to the neurological specialist who has treated me for over 10 years. My complex neurological disease—5 brain surgeries, 3 spinal surgeries and a rare diagnoses [sp]—was in the hands of an Ob/Gyn. Let that sink in.

Strategies and tactics to deny patient care! It's never a peer and it's never a review.[8]

Then she mentioned the CEO of her insurance company, listed his salary—$22.1 million—and tagged him, the badass that she is.

Ultimately, she won her expedited appeal and she's back on IVIG and feeling more like herself again.[ii] She could have stopped at

---

[ii] As of early 2026, Sally was once again fighting her insurance company, who deemed her IVIG treatments no longer "medically necessary." Sally won and coverage of her treatments resumed.

her own personal victory, but she wanted to make sure that other patients didn't have to go through the same ordeal. That meant taking on the politicians who have sway in how health insurance works or doesn't work.

"I never wanted to dabble in politics in any way ever. But here I am, knee deep in the shit. Pardon the French." That *shit* is her work as a self-trained patient advocate, which ultimately led to her conversations with Senator Bernie Sanders' office and testimony at her state capitol in North Carolina, where two physician lawmakers introduced a bipartisan prior authorization reform bill in 2025.

"I jumped in with two feet and started talking to all of the representatives in North Carolina," she recalled. The bill passed and is now acting as a blueprint for other states to introduce similar legislation.

Nix reports hearing stories daily from patients like her who have had to battle their own health insurance companies for coverage. She fights for them because the system fights against them.

"Laws are changing, so [health insurance companies] are going to figure out another way. There's always a loophole with them." It has so inspired Sally that she's a co-founder of We the Patients (see Chapter 9), and we're lucky to have her ideas and her chutzpah on board with us.

No wonder patients are so pissed that some of them even threw money and social media support behind the likes of Luigi Mangione.[iii] His extreme actions, which his manifesto referred to as "brutal honesty," may have become a catalyst for health insurance reform. As he pointed out, America has the most expensive healthcare system in the world and yet, in 2025, our life expectancy ranked forty-eighth,[9] about four years shorter than in other developed countries (Figure 2.2). That's an entire presidential administration less. Is our system worth it?

[iii]Reminder: murder = bad.

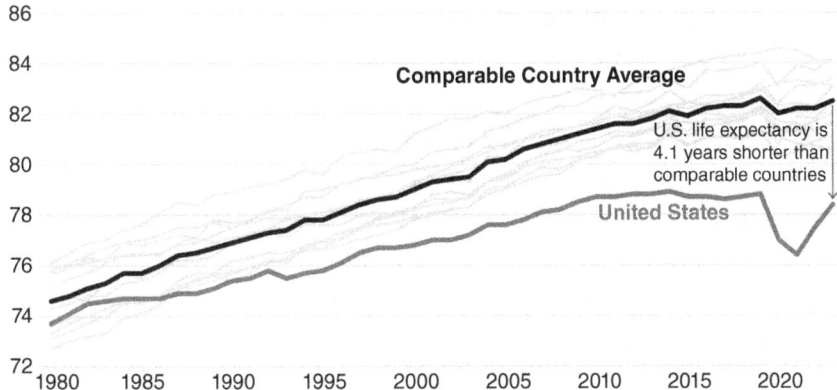

FIGURE 2.2 Life Expectancy at Birth, 1980–2023. Notes: Comparable countries include Australia, Austria, Belgium, Canada, France, Germany, Japan, the Netherlands, Sweden, Switzerland, and the United Kingdom. 2023 UK life expectancy data is only for England and Wales. See Methods section of "How does U.S. life expectancy compare to other countries?" Source: Peterson-KFF Health System Tracker, https://www.healthsystemtracker.org/chart-collection/u-s-life-expectancy-compare-countries

The "P" Word

We spend the most, but we don't necessarily get the best. Our convoluted healthcare system, which often pits patients against profits, is set up to squeeze as much money as possible from the healthcare process, and it starts with prior authorizations, when your insurance company determines whether or not they'll cover a test, procedure, or treatment. Or as the American Medical Association (AMA) calls them, "a barrier to providing timely, patient-centered care."[10]

But tell us how you really feel, docs.

Prior authorizations delay care while your doctor is forced to justify their medical decisions and you wait around to find out the verdict, like a tribute in *The Hunger Games*. What happens when your prior auth gets the thumbs-down? It's pretty common, occurring about a quarter of the time, says the American Medical Association (AMA),[11] and increasingly, a robot is making that decision, using artificial intelligence to supply speedy batch denials. The lightning-fast process of about a second means that insurance companies can now deny prior auths that used to cost them more to review by human doctors,[12] who are slower. And robots don't feel the tiniest bit bad about telling you that your healthcare isn't "medically necessary."

In 2024, the AMA asked doctors how prior authorizations affected patients in their care. The results were alarming:

- Some 93 percent of doctors reported care delays while patients awaited approval.
- More than a quarter reported that prior auths led to a serious adverse event for a patient in their care.
- Doctors and their staff spend an average of thirteen hours a week completing prior auths.
- About a third reported that their prior auths are often or always denied.[13]

Like most healthcare industry shenanigans, prior authorizations started out small, and then when they started to pad wallets, they were expanded. Originally called "utilization reviews," they were designed to control hospital admission costs when Medicare and Medicaid were babies back in the 1960s. The goal was to avoid the "overutilization of resources and identify waste."[14] In other words, they acted as a stopgap for treatment that could be administered in outpatient (and therefore, much less expensive) settings.

Private health insurance companies liked the model so much, they began reviewing claims for "medical necessity" through a prior authorization process,[15] yada, yada, and now we have robots denying healthcare claims. We went from "doctors know best" to artificial intelligence having a say in who gets healthcare.

Prior authorizations may have been designed to reduce waste, but they've actually *added* costs to the healthcare system, leading to additional doctor's office visits, increased ER admissions and hospitalizations, and "step therapy," when patients are forced to try and fail other less expensive treatments before the one prescribed by the doctor is approved. Or not.[16]

If you think that a prior authorization is the golden ticket to care, you must be from another country or you've never used your American health insurance. Healthcare.org describes it this way: *"Prior authorization is not a guarantee that a claim will be approved, but failure to obtain prior authorization for a service that requires it will generally result in a claim denial."*[17]

It's like your parents telling you that it's okay to take the car tonight to go to the movies with friends and then later punishing you for taking the car. I don't get it. I really don't. How can an insurance company approve a test, a medication, or a treatment and then say, "JK, no it's not" after you've already incurred the cost? Through claim denial, when an insurance company refuses to pay for a service or medication despite prior authorization.

Welcome to America.

Your Responsibility

While prior authorizations cause delays and can lead to denials of care, that's all happening before a service is provided or a medication is prescribed. Claim denial, when your insurance company refuses to cover costs for a procedure or treatment you've already gotten, can leave patients holding the bill.

You have the surgery or get the chemo or the infusions and then your insurance company says, "Not our problem." Next, your Explanation of Benefits (EOB), that list of what's covered and what's not, ends up with four-, five-, six-, even seven-figure dollar amounts under the words "Your Responsibility." It's enough to make you sick.

Healthcare insurance companies deny, on average, up to 20 percent[18] of claims, though some of the biggies (*cough, cough,* UnitedHealthcare) reject an average of about a third[19] of all claims. KFF identified the most common reasons for claim denials:

- lack of prior authorization or referral
- out-of-network provider
- exclusion of a service (it's not covered by your plan)
- medical necessity (as determined by a doctor hired by your insurance company)
- all other reasons[20]

Three-quarters of denials make up "all other reasons"[21] and they can create some confusing and confounding EOBs. (Side note: No other industry reveals the price *after* the work is done.) Many of the denials have nothing to do with you or your health. They include mistakes made by whoever's filling out the claim, such as incorrect or missing coding, late filing, misspellings, and incorrect policy numbers, or exceeding coverage limits (i.e., 10 physical therapy sessions were okayed, but you submitted 12). Sometimes it has to do with coverage, like a procedure or an expensive treatment that's not covered by your plan or a doctor who's out-of-network.

Perhaps one of the highest-profile examples of the state of insurance denials happened during one of Dr. Elisabeth Potter's breast reconstruction DIEP flap surgeries. The Austin, Texas-based surgeon said that UnitedHealthcare called after her patient had been put under anesthesia in the OR. Worried that the insurance company might deny the surgery it had already approved, thereby leaving her patient with an enormous bill, she took the call. Turns out, it was about the in-patient overnight stay, as she reported on Instagram in a post that instantly went viral:

"I had to scrub out mid-surgery to call United[Healthcare], only to find that the person on the line didn't even have access to the patient's full medical information, despite the procedure already being pre-approved."[22]

Weeks later, she received a letter from UnitedHealthcare's law firm demanding she remove the video from social media and post an apology.[23] Dr. Potter told *The Times* that UnitedHealthcare has since refused to provide in-network coverage of her surgery center, and she's set up a GoFundMe fundraiser.[24] As she said in her viral video, "Insurance is out of control. I have no other words."

Dr. Potter isn't the only person pushing back on delays and denials by health insurance companies. In 2023, two plaintiffs filed a class action complaint in the United States District Court in Minnesota against UnitedHealthcare alleging the "illegal deployment of artificial intelligence in place of real medical professionals to wrongfully deny elderly patients care owed to them." They said the Defendants knew that the AI model used for denials had a 90 percent error rate. "Defendants bank on the patients' impaired conditions, lack of knowledge, and lack of resources to appeal the erroneous AI-powered decisions."[25]

As of this writing, the class action is proceeding. But we can't all be plaintiffs or badass patient advocates in scrubs, and we shouldn't have to be. Yet the healthcare system isn't getting easier to navigate.

About three-quarters of Americans, across demographic groups, income levels, and political parties, find the delay and denial tactics used by health insurance companies to be troublesome, reports *KFF Health*.[26] Finally, something we can all come together on: We don't want to die on hold while on the phone with our health insurance companies.

Yet few step up even to fight for themselves. Health insurance claim appeals by patients are exceptionally rare, accounting for just 0.2 percent of denied claims. There are some 73 million in-network claims denied each year[27] (Figure 2.3), and most of us just shut up and take it.

And that's just the healthcare idiocracy that most people have heard about. Wait until you find out about what's likely happening at your pharmacy.

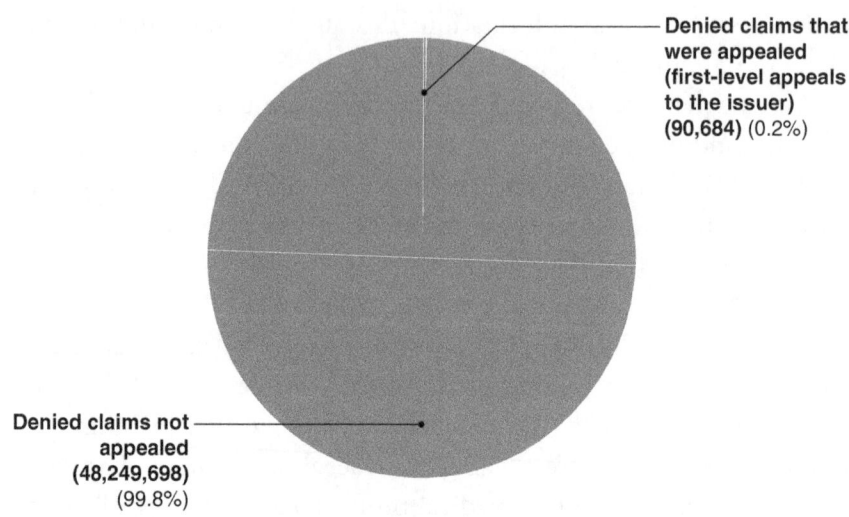

FIGURE 2.3   Consumers Rarely Appeal Denied Health Insurance Claims. Note: This figure only includes denied claims for issuers that show data on appealed claims.
Source: Karen Pollitz, Justin Lo, Rayna Wallace, and Salem Mengistu, "Claims Denials and Appeals in ACA Marketplace Plans in 2021," KFF, February 9, 2023. Available at: https://www.kff.org/private-insurance/claims-denials-and-appeals-in-aca-marketplace-plans/

Enter the Middlemen

Between 2016 and 2023, denials for prescription drugs rose by 25 percent,[28] and many of the denials didn't even come directly from insurance companies, but from Pharmacy Benefit Managers (PBMs), intermediaries who negotiate drug prices and manage lists of covered medications called formularies, for millions of Americans. Sounds reasonable and maybe even helpful, right? Please hold while the system screws this up, too.

Like most everything involved in modern American healthcare, PBMs started as a simple idea that eventually became tangled up in the system. It began with an increased demand for prescription drugs. The 1960s was an era of pharma breakthroughs, including major blood-pressure drugs and blood thinners.[29] The first birth control pill hit the market, and there were 58 million new prescriptions and nearly twice as many refills for sedatives and tranquilizers,[30] which might explain why the Rolling Stones' "Mother's Little Helper" was such a hit.

At the same time, the government took on some of the burden for healthcare and prescription costs through the newly minted Medicare and Medicaid programs. In 1967, the Johnson administration's Task Force on Prescription Drugs calculated that the cost of out-of-hospital prescription drugs had risen dramatically as the number of Rxs per person nearly doubled, from 2.4 to 4.75. That was expensive, especially for the elderly, with costs rising from $736 million in 1950 to a whopping $3.25 billion in 1967.[31]

But back then, people often paid out-of-pocket for their prescriptions. Over the decades, insurers increasingly picked up the tab or at least part of it. Health plans, big employers, unions, and the government started contracting third-party administrators called PBMs to manage their drug benefits programs.[32] Working on behalf of health insurance companies, PBMs processed prescription drug claims. In time, their role expanded to include setting drug formularies and co-pays and having a hand in prior authorizations and pharmacy choice.[33] If you can only get a second-choice drug to the one your doctor prescribed and you have to go to a pharmacy that's not yours to get it, thank a PBM.

Then in 2003, Congress passed the Medicare Modernization Act, which added coverage for prescription drugs through Part D. This gave PBMs a bigger role in handling the paperwork, setting drug pricing, and negotiating discounts and rebates.[34] Today, the three biggest PBMs,

CVS Caremark, Express Scripts, and UnitedHealthcare's OptumRx, account for 80 percent of the market.[35]

So what's the problem? As the Pharmacists Society of the State of New York put it, the PBM business model "masquerades as a 'cost saver,' but is actually a cost multiplier,"[36] with PBMs taking their cut of the cash at every stage of the process. Here's how:

- **Spread pricing:** PBMs charge insurers one price for drugs and reimburse pharmacies at a lower price, pocketing the difference.[37]
- **Maximum Allowable Cost (MAC):** One way they do that is by setting the MAC, the highest price allowable for generic drugs and brand name drugs that have generics available. PBMs then "reimburse low and charge high with their MAC price lists, pocketing the significant spread between the two prices."[38]
- **DIR fees:** The idea, which arose from the Medicare Modernization Act, was for PBMs to administer Medicare Part D plans and in turn, collect "direct and indirect reimbursement" (DIR) fees for the effort. PBMs then "claw back" a fee from the pharmacy after the fact, cutting the pharmacy's profits by as much as 50 percent. In one example from a report commissioned by the Community Oncology Alliance, a 5 percent DIR fee for a $2,000 cancer drug lines the PBM's pocket by $100 for each Rx.[39] *Newsweek* reports, "Cancer medications are already expensive, and now PBMs are imposing an additional fee calculated as a percentage of the cost of that pricey drug."[40]
- **Administration fees:** This is like Ticketmaster, but for prescription drugs—fees and payments that are part of the cost of transacting with a PBM. But as Affirmed Rx, a PBM that claims to offer transparency and patient-centric care, explained, "Even the savviest of employers cannot typically understand the various charges they are paying due to complex drug contracting."[41] These fees drive up the cost of your meds, and especially impact people with high-deductible plans, reports Affirmed Rx.

- **Vertical integration:** Ever wonder who owns PBMs? Quite possibly, your own health insurance company. Some of the largest PBMs are owned by health insurers:

PBM	Parent Organization
CVS Caremark	CVS Health with Aetna
EnvisionRx	Rite Aid
Envolve Rx	Centene Corporation
Evernorth	Cigna
Express Scripts	Cigna
Humana Pharmacy Solutions	Humana
Kaiser Permanente PBM	Kaiser Permanente
Optum Rx	UnitedHealth Group
Prime Therapeutics	Blue Cross/Blue Shield

- **Rebates:** PBMs have a built-in incentive to skim money from the process, says the American Economic Liberties Project. That's because PBMs run the formularies, the list of drugs sold at a pharmacy. "To gain more favorable formulary placement, drug manufacturers will offer discounts to PBMs in the form of 'rebates' that the manufacturer pays to the PBM, who then pays the insurance company," Zach Freed wrote for the American Economic Liberties Project in an article about what he called, "the pharmacy benefit mafia." But PBMs are exempt from anti-kickback statutes under Medicare, so they take a cut.[42]

If you're wondering who's allowing PBMs to behave like Ray Liotta's Henry Hill in *Goodfellas*—"Business bad? Fuck you, pay me"— start with your state government. Most state-level laws designed to curb PBM practices have failed after the Federal Trade Commission (FTC) sent letters to local legislators in California, New Jersey, New York, North Dakota, Rhode Island, and Virginia, discouraging them from doing so in the 2000s.[43]

The FTC finally stepped up in 2024 to sue the top three PBMs, alleging that they abused their economic power by using a "perverse" system and "rigging pharmaceutical supply chain competition in their favor, forcing patients to pay more for life-saving medication."[44]

There are simply too few effective efforts to protect patients and too many working against our best interests.

Playing Politics

Why are we letting this happen? Ask your lawmakers. In Chapter 1, I showed you America's century-long struggle with healthcare reform. But if I had to pinpoint the precise moment we lost the plot and drove the story to our current chaotic situation, I'd rewind the videotape to 1993, when President Bill Clinton delivered an address about his healthcare reform proposal on live national television. He said, "It is time for America to fix a healthcare system that's badly broken."[45] Then he said many of the things that get supporters of healthcare reform excited that someone's finally going to step up and make some real, lasting changes to help all Americans, especially those of us who use a lot of healthcare:

- "Millions of Americans are just a pink slip away from losing their healthcare coverage, and one serious illness away from losing their life savings."[46] *Preach, Bill!*
- "I believe that Medicare should cover the cost of prescription drugs."[47] *No brainer.*
- "The proposal I will describe tonight will reform the costliest and the most wasteful healthcare system on Earth without any broad-based taxes."[48] *Oh, if only that were true.*

His plan included a "healthcare security card" that would guarantee coverage for all Americans. It didn't matter if you left your job and, therefore, your healthcare coverage, to start your own business, or if you retired before sixty-five, or if you had a pre-existing condition. With this card, everyone could get healthcare. The plan prohibited insurance companies from dropping you for getting sick, and it provided coverage for all the greatest healthcare hits, from doctor's appointments to hospital visits to preventative screening. It was as though Canada had dropped by and left behind its healthcare system.

In "The Clinton Health Plan Is Alive On Arrival," *The New York Times* gushed about the Clintons' plan, telling the story of how Hillary, who spearheaded the effort, had "dazzled" Congressional committees. But it also introduced an opponent to the story, Rep. Newt Gingrich (R-GA) who promised a full-blast assault on the Clinton plan over costs and his view that government, at its core, is inept. "The bureaucracy that can't get the right speech in the Teleprompter can't get the right CAT scan to the doctor, either."[49]

Oh, crap. I hope this guy doesn't get power . . . oh, that's right. Gingrich would become the Speaker of the House after the GOP's midterm takeover in 1994 and serve as the brains behind The Contract with America, which railed against big government.[50] As Harvard professor Theda Skocpol would later write, "Toward the end of 1993, right-wing Republicans realized that their ideological fortunes within their own party, as well as the Republican partisan interest in weakening the Democrats as a prelude to winning control of Congress and the presidency, could be splendidly served by first demonizing and then totally defeating the Clinton plan."[51]

When the Clintons' task force started working on their healthcare reform plan in late 1993, Americans approved of it by a two-to-one margin.[52] By June 1994, however, support had plummeted to about a third.[53] It was a midterm election year, and the opposition bombarded the public with dire warnings of the "welfarization of healthcare," which is an actual headline by Gingrich and Rep. Dick Armey (R-TX) in the *National Review*. They wrote, "If you like the way the Federal Government runs public housing and the state government runs the Department of Motor Vehicles, you'll love healthcare under the Clinton Plan."[54]

Critics on the right started calling the plan "Hillarycare" in opposition messaging in editorials and on conservative talk radio shows to capitalize on the right's disdain for the First Lady. Princeton professor Paul Starr wrote in *The American Prospect* that while focus groups approved the healthcare reform plan at a rate of 70 percent, when it had a Clinton name in the title, approval dropped by up to forty points.[55] (It's just like when your aunt doesn't want "that Obamacare" when she's already got it. It's the ACA. Politicians deliberately use words to confuse and influence us.)

There were multiple reasons the plan tanked, but it was the opposition's master class in divisive messaging that ultimately shepherded it to its death. After George Will wrote in *Newsweek* that the plan would make it illegal for doctors to accept money directly from patients outside of a government health plan, the idea of "doctors in jail" started showing up on talk shows for the rest of the year.[56] Political Action Committees (PACs) threw money behind those anti-Clinton health plan "Harry and Louise" ads (see Chapter 1) sponsored by insurance associations,[57] and soon, people started carrying protest signs that riffed on Bon Jovi, "ClintonCare is Bad Medicine."[58]

Conservative radio host Rush Limbaugh said, "I don't have time to beat around the bush. The healthcare plan as proposed by Mrs. Clinton is socialism." And there it was. The S-word that had torpedoed so many healthcare reform plans throughout the century. Other columnists began throwing it around, too, and voila! We were right back where we always wind up when it comes to any hint of universal healthcare in America: DOA.

In Skocpol's lecture, aptly titled, "The Time is Never Ripe: The Repeated Defeat of Universal Health Insurance in the 20th Century United States," she declared, "Very possibly, Americans who favor governmentally mediated universal health insurance have just had— and lost—their last opportunity for achieving it."[59]

It wasn't exactly the last though. The Clintons would set the stage for another Democrat to try to give us healthcare options that aren't tied to employment when President Obama introduced the ACA in 2009. That one would stick for a long time, but boy, would it take a lot of hits.

A Swing and a Miss

Before we get to Obamacare, we must take a detour through the Patients' Bill of Rights legislation of 2001. Excuse me, the *bipartisan* legislation, introduced by Senators McCain (R-AZ), Kennedy (D-MA), and Edwards (D-NC) in the Senate and by Rep. Ganske (R-IA), Dingell (D-MI), and Norwood (R-GA) in the House of Representatives. It even had President George W. Bush's support. Well, sort of.

The bill would provide patient protections for every American enrolled in a health plan. As *Managed Healthcare Executive* explained in the early days of this century, "In October, 1999, the House had approved a sweeping measure that would have guaranteed patients a long list of powers over their health plans, including the right to seek reimbursed care in the nearest emergency department, to see specialists outside the plan if the plan did not have one signed up and, for women, to see an OB/GYN without a referral."[60]

It passed the Senate. It eked through the Republican-controlled House with changes urged by President Bush, including scaling back lawsuits against HMOs that the Senate version would have allowed.[61] And then it, too, got killed in reconciliation, where both chambers have to come to an agreement on their versions of the bill.

In time, at least thirty states passed their own versions of patients' rights legislation, which includes statutes that ensure access to specialists and ER care. Some states even have liability statutes that allow lawsuits for wrongful denials of healthcare coverage.

Then in 2010, a federal Patient Bill of Rights showed up again, in the Affordable Care Act, but it didn't provide the lawsuit rights. Yet its other protections included the kind of things that the Clintons could only dream of.

I Got It on the Exchange

The ACA isn't and never was universal healthcare, but it has provided many people with affordable-ish healthcare coverage that they couldn't get before and some pretty cool patient protections.

For some people, these were nice little perks should they ever lose their jobs and therefore, their health insurance. But for others, it was like Oprah shouting, "And you get healthcare! And you get healthcare! And you, too!" Unfortunately, the opposition felt the same way, as though they'd unwillingly taken on Oprah's role as the funder in this analogy, and they set out to take it down—dozens and dozens of times.

For those of us in cancer advocacy, the single most important victory of Obamacare was eliminating pre-existing conditions as a variable for individual healthcare coverage. A quarter of adults under age 65 reportedly have a pre-existing health condition,[62] and the US Department of Health and Human Services (HHS) estimated that half of all adult Americans had some sort of pre-existing condition, from asthma to diabetes to cancer. The HHS said in 2011: "Without the Affordable Care Act, such conditions limit the ability to obtain affordable health insurance if they become self-employed, take a job with a company that does not offer coverage, or experience a change in life circumstance, such as divorce, retirement, or moving to a different state."[63]

If you didn't have a job at a giant corporation with great health insurance, a cancer diagnosis could have wiped you out financially. The ACA made it economically safer for the self-employed, divorced, retired before 65, and others to get sick and sicker. It also made it illegal for your insurer to kick you off your plan if you got sick.

It provided other very important protections as well:

- Coverage for children up to age 26
- Ending lifetime and annual dollar limits on "essential health benefits"
- Providing free preventive care[64]
- Keeping insurers from varying their rates based on your health condition or gender[65]
- Preventing your insurer from requiring higher co-pays if you go to an out-of-network ER

- Preventing insurers from being able to cancel your coverage just because your employer made a mistake on your insurance application.[66] Yes, you read that right. Before the ACA, if Karen in HR accidentally listed your birthdate wrong, or whatever, your insurance "could take away your coverage, declare your policy invalid, and ask you to pay back any money they had spent on your medical care."[67]

Was the ACA perfect? No. Remember President Obama's promise, "If you like your doctor, you can keep your doctor"? Yeah, not really true. In 2013, PolitiFact labeled this claim a "pants on fire,"[68] which sounds like it could use an ambulance ride. I hope it's covered.

But Obamacare has provided more than 40 million people with health insurance, dropping the uninsured rate from 14.5 percent in 2013 to 8.6 percent within three years.[69] How the heck did it pass when the Clintons couldn't get their version over the finish line?

First, they didn't pass it down from the president on "stone tablets," as Obama's political adviser David Axelrod put it, instead turning to Congress to create their own plan.[70] They didn't start from scratch. Congress modeled the plan after Republican Mitt Romney's successful plan in Massachusetts.[71] Yes, I said Mitt Romney. Look it up. They originally based it on an individual mandate that required everyone to get healthcare coverage, with subsidies for those who needed it and Medicaid for the poor.[72]

This last part rankled small government-loving lawmakers, but it didn't kill the bill.

In 2009, the Democrats had the largest Senate majority since the eighties, so they had the numbers to pass it. Even so, the bill got stuck in the Finance Committee. No worries, because House Speaker Nancy Pelosi was relentless when it came to Obamacare. The House started its own bill and she helped push it through, pulling out the stops on her negotiating (read: guilting and pressuring) skills.

But of course, Republicans in both the Senate and the House began their assault, spreading rumors of "death panels" deciding if your grandma would get healthcare to keep her alive, railing about abortion coverage, and insisting that undocumented immigrants would be covered by our tax dollars. When Obama took on these issues in an address to Congress after Senator Ted Kennedy's death from a brain tumor, Rep. Joe Wilson (R-SC) shouted, "You lie!"[73]

The Senate could pass the bill as long as no Dems voted against it, and they pulled it off. Though the House bill was unpopular—its price tag was a trillion bucks—and moderate Dems walked out of negotiations over reimbursements, it passed 219–212, with zero GOP votes.[74] In Pelosi's closing speech, she said, "We will be joining those who established Social Security, Medicare, and now, tonight, healthcare for all Americans."[75]

Now, how can America ruin this? Let me count the ways: 70. At least 70.

Weaken, Defund, Repeal

Each and every Congress since the ACA passed has introduced legislation to weaken, defund, or repeal it. The opposition said that the ACA drove up healthcare costs and prevented small businesses from hiring, and they wanted to return "patient choice" to the system. Here are their greatest hits:

2011

The GOP took control of the House of Representatives and got right down to the businesses of attacking the ACA. They introduced a bill called "Repealing the Job-Killing Health Care Law Act."[76] Obama said he'd veto whatever came through, and it died.

2012

Even after the Supreme Court upheld the ACA as constitutional, the GOP held a vote in the house to repeal it and all the Republicans and five Democrats voted yes, but it failed to pass the Senate and of course,

Obama would have canned it anyhow. Or as ABC News' "House Obamacare Repeal: Thirty-Third Time's the Charm?" put it, "There is not a snowball's chance that this repeal will be signed into law."[77]

2013

While Democrats held the Senate, the Republicans, led by Speaker John Boehner, maintained the House. In late 2013, the federal government shut down, and the GOP tried to use it as a way to dismantle the ACA, including a 21-hour, Senate floor, filibuster-style speech by Ted Cruz (R-TX) during which he equated the fight against supplying Americans with healthcare with the battle against Nazis and read from Dr. Seuss' "Green Eggs and Ham."[78] Senate Democratic Leader Harry Reid called it "a big waste of time." In the end, which was sixteen days later, it was a bad look for the Republicans, who backed down, and the ACA came out unscathed.[79] For now.

2015

The Republicans gained control of both the House and the Senate for the first time since George W. Bush was in office. The House passed the Restoring Americans' Healthcare Freedom Reconciliation Act of 2015 in an attempt to repeal the ACA altogether, targeting many of the fundamentals of Obamacare, including the individual mandate that required all Americans to have health insurance, Medicaid expansion funding, and subsidies.[80] An amended version passed the House and then President Obama vetoed it. The Congressional Budget Office (CBO) meanwhile reported that the plan would have kicked 18 million people off insurance and that by 2026, 32 million would have become uninsured.[81]

2017

The Republicans took control of the White House, the Senate, and the House—the trifecta. They wasted no time coming after Obamacare. President Donald Trump signed an executive order to expand insurance options for Americans beyond the ACA to association health plans that, unlike many ACA plans, cross state lines. Their ideas came with a cost to patients. Former Obama official Andy Slavitt told *The Wall Street Journal*, "Its aim is clearly to do with the pen what Congress wouldn't—eliminate pre-existing condition protections, essential benefit protections, and lifetime caps, and turn the ACA into a sparsely available high-risk pool."[82]

Throughout the year, various bills were introduced to sink the ACA by repealing individual and employer mandates, canning tax credits, and reducing Medicaid expansion through "Trumpcare."[83] It passed the House, but a pared down "skinny repeal" version died by a 49–51 vote on the Senate floor when Senator John McCain (R-AZ), dying of brain cancer, famously gave a late-night thumbs-down vote.

At the time, President Trump tweeted, "3 Republicans and 48 Democrats let the American people down. As I said from the beginning, let Obamacare implode, then deal. Watch!"[84] Which is an easy thing to say when you have presidential-level healthcare for life and no known brain tumors.

It's not that McCain championed Obamacare. He said the Senate legislation was a "shell of a bill" that didn't go far enough to increase competition, lower costs, and improve healthcare."[85] In the end—he died less than a year later—his vote wasn't about supporting the ACA at all. It was about following procedure in the Senate, despite campaign promises.[86] So our protections against getting booted off our insurance for a cancer diagnosis was ultimately preserved by one senator's dedication to Congressional protocol.[87] This time.

2018

A collection of red states filed a lawsuit in a Texas district court seeking to invalidate the ACA as unconstitutional over the individual mandate.[88] In 2021, the Supreme Court said the plaintiffs lacked standing and threw it out of court.

By 2020, attacks against the ACA slowed, and the cease fire continued into President Joe "Cancer Moonshot" Biden's term in office. I guess it's hard to get support for wiping out people's healthcare during a global pandemic. In fact, the ACA had its biggest approval rating in 2020, with 55 percent of Americans favoring Obamacare, and that was in February, just before the COVID-19 shutdown, before millions of people began losing their jobs and, therefore, their health insurance.[89]

For fifteen years, Obamacare survived, even when there was a Republican-controlled Congress and White House. In all, there were about 70 attempts at repeal, and though they didn't kill it, the ACA still took on shrapnel along the way.

Remember, the ACA is not one cohesive American health plan. It is fifty different systems, each with its own collection of rules and laws. Before Trump's second term, several states scaled back Medicaid coverage or added work requirements and reduced access for emergency care coverage for undocumented immigrants. Meanwhile, provider networks in the ACA narrowed so that healthcare consumers had fewer choices of plans and doctors, all while premiums rose quickly—50 percent faster than employer health plans.[90]

It was like the ACA had become the Black Knight in "Monty Python and the Holy Grail," sliced and diced down, all the while insisting, "Tis but a scratch." Then in 2025, with the Republicans holding power of both the White House and Congress once again, they came in for the kill with the One Big Beautiful Bill (OBBB). This time, they brought a chainsaw.

One Big Beautiful Bill

Though President Trump's One Big Beautiful Bill, signed into law on July 4, 2025, because 'Murica, wasn't specifically a direct attack on the ACA, it was designed to weaken it, not to mention Medicaid. It shortened the enrollment period and cut enhanced tax credits.[91]

The CBO estimated that more than three million people would become uninsured because of the ACA provisions alone, and taken together with cuts to Medicaid, some 16 million people would end up uninsured into the next decade.[92]

As of this writing months after the bill became law, it has already pushed ACA premiums higher in several states, with 11 states experiencing rate increases exceeding 30 percent.[93] Rural hospitals are warning about service cuts or permanent closure. Federal analysts are outlining scenarios where Medicare—yes MediCARE—trims benefits for the first time in its history. The country feels unstable and the ground keeps shifting under the people who need care the most.

By the time you read this page the landscape may look even stranger. Maybe America has slid into a Mad Max-style version of healthcare where roaming bands of angry patients in hospital gowns, lugging IV poles and fighting over the last Jell-O in the fridge.

I haven't even covered all the ways healthcare chicanery works against us. Don't forget the excessive-to-outrageous price of medications and hospitalizations that somehow keep increasing, the ubiquitous medical bankruptcies, and the disheartening cuts to cancer research funding. But you get the gist.

If you feel like all is lost and you want to put on some hospital socks and a robe and go curl up in a ball, I know exactly what that is like. I navigated this system back when it was far less humane and I was just a kid. Then I dusted myself off and worked with other like-minded advocates to make it better for us all.

3 We the Survivors

The summer before my senior year of college in 1995, I started getting wicked headaches. I was a classically trained pianist studying to become a film composer, and I had one more year before grad school at the University of Southern California, where I'd study with the late, great, Jerry Goldsmith. I was just twenty-one, but I knew exactly what I wanted to do with the rest of my life.

That's when the fuckery began.

I had the privilege of working as a tech intern at Dean Witter Reynolds in Tower Two of the World Trade Center. I was hired through a temp agency to manage the company's scores of printers across multiple floors. Basically, I was the "toner guy," the kid who unjammed paper and made sure the printers were connected to the "intranet." (Look it up, kids.)

I started getting headaches, subtle and gradual, until mid-summer when they became downright horrible. But I chalked up the vertigo I was experiencing to the express elevators, powered by what I called "flux capacitors," hoist motors shooting me up to the sixty-eighth floor every morning. I figured it was a New York City–specific occupational hazard.

But these headaches weren't like the front-of-the-head kind you get after too much tequila or the first spoonful of ice cream. The pain was coming from the back left part of my head, behind the ear and near my neck.

I popped some Tylenol and kept on working.

When I returned to school that fall, the pain got worse. My brain felt like it was in a slow-press waffle iron. I had a hard time arpeggiating, which is when you play piano notes in a progression, with my dominant left hand. I assumed that I hadn't practiced enough over the summer, so I doubled down and rehearsed more. Cue the Rocky-style training montage. But it didn't help. A month later, I was trying to sign a credit card receipt at a cash register at the mall, but I couldn't hold the pen, so my friend signed it for me. We didn't think anything of it.

But I just wasn't feeling right, so I kept going back to the campus doctor that semester. First, he diagnosed me with carpal tunnel syndrome and told me to sling my backpack on the other shoulder. The next time I went, he called it Epstein–Barr syndrome and prescribed rest. Next up: early onset multiple sclerosis, then maybe a stroke, and finally, the flu. He gave me Robitussin cough syrup and told me to take it easy.

By midterms, I'd lost around 25 percent of the fine motor skills in my left hand. I could barely hold a pen to write music, and I failed a music history test simply because I couldn't write fast enough. I even had a hard time opening doors and picking things up. I began to have dizzy spells and moments of "zoning out," when I'd just stare off into the distance. The headaches, meanwhile, had become blood-curdling. If I had to describe the pain by picking one of the face emojis on a pain-scale chart, which range from smiley to sad, I would have drawn in Edvard Munch's "The Scream."

I decided that the best remedy was to work harder. I had a massive thirty-credit course-load, along with theatrical performances, once even managing to play the piano in the pit using just my right hand. What can I say? I was young and I felt invincible.

By mid-November, though, I'd become a train wreck. The head-aches were now crippling. I couldn't grip a pen or use my dominant left hand for anything, so I brought my laptop to class, back when no one did and there was no such thing as Wi-Fi, pecking my notes with my right pointer finger on the very-cool-for-the-times Power-Book 180 or my Macintosh Centris 650 with a color monitor. Only, my music professor thought—and I am being entirely serious here—that I was "beaming answers from space." Even if I could, there was nothing on what passed for the internet in 1995 that could have been remotely helpful with Music History 401.

By late November, I had two musicals to produce as music direc-tor: *Joseph and the Amazing Technicolor Dreamcoat* and Edwin Gorey's *Gorey Stories*. I just kept working around the parts of my body that weren't functioning too well.

Somehow, I packed up some stuff and drove home for Thanksgiv-ing break. When I told my parents about my symptoms, they right-fully lost their shit. They were so pissed that I hadn't bothered to tell them anything about it over the course of the semester, even though I was a good Jewish son and called home regularly. They set up an appointment with my pediatrician; at twenty-one, I didn't yet have a GP. He recommended some tests.

"Can this wait until after the semester ends?" I asked. "I've got two musicals to produce plus about six final exams and papers to write."

And my doctor replied, "Sure."

Sure. I had screaming headaches, I'd all but lost the use of my dominant hand, I had vertigo, and I would lose my balance just walk-ing across the room. But sure, go ahead and finish up your course load, kid.

Just one day after I returned to school in early December, I was on the phone in my dorm room and suddenly, I slurred one of my words. It was as if my mouth went numb. And *that* was when it finally hit me how serious this was. I knew I was careening down-hill toward a Very Bad Neighborhood, and yet, I had stuff to do, so I kept this new and alarming symptom to myself while my teachers and friends told me what anyone would say when a young person is sick:

"It's probably nothing."
"You need a few nights of good sleep."
"Just take a vacation and you'll be fine."
"It's all in your head." (Ironic, eh?)

I finished my shows and my finals and then I called my dad, and, in a moment of clarity, I told him I was too compromised to drive home for the break. At the end of the semester, he drove up, helped me pack my things, and drove me home.

During the last two weeks of December, all the shit hit the fan for me. It was like a movie scene where the cop is shooting at the bad guy but he Just. Won't. Die. Bullet after bullet, he keeps walking on and on. That was me. Slurred speech? I'll keep trying to speak. Double vision? One of those images is the right one. Lightheadedness, fainting, trouble walking? No worries. I'll just get back up again and keep going.

Concerned, my mom took me back to the pediatrician, who, this time, took my litany of symptoms very seriously, recommending an EEG. I was so nervous at the neurologist's visit, I puked on him. Though he found nothing else awry, he recommended an MRI. My father would write in his journal, "I felt in my heart it was a tumor!"

When we got home from the scan, the answering machine light was blinking, signaling we had a message—a message we instinctively knew was not good. The doctor wanted me to come back for more tests because there was something in my brain.

Essentially, I was diagnosed over an answering machine.

We returned for a second MRI, this time with gadolinium, a contrast agent that Dr. Google says is "toxic to humans." Then we found out how not good it was: The Chief of Neurosurgery, who was an Orthodox Jew, wanted to meet us the next day, a Friday, the Sabbath. That's when I knew I'd arrived at the Welcome Center for a Very Bad Neighborhood.

And meet us, he did. Every patient should have a moment—for us that Friday, it was three hours of moments—like this with their doctor. He explained everything he knew at that point: I had a golf ball-sized mass in my brain, but we wouldn't know if it's cancer until the pathology report came in. I'd need surgery and possibly radiation. Maybe chemo. They were going to do whatever it took to make me better.

When the pathology report came in, we discovered the hard truth: I had cancer. All my docs thought it was a pilocytic astrocytoma, a low-grade brain tumor that typically gets better with treatment. But the slides showed a more concerning diagnosis: a congenital medulloblastoma, an aggressive type of cancer with a less optimistic prognosis.

My "Uncle Jay," who was my godfather and my dad's best friend since junior high school in Bensonhurst back in the fifties, happened to be a world-renowned geneticist. He sent my pathology slides to the top geneticists and pathologists around the world. He came back a week later with confirmation that it was indeed a medulloblastoma, which, back then, was classified as a rare PNET, a primitive neuro-ectodermal tumor.

No one could believe it, including my surgeon. Medulloblastomas are all automatically classified as Grade IV, and there is no Grade V. The kind I had is a fast-growing bastard with the ability to turn deadly within months. When it runs out of room in your head, it can drop little cancer cell seeds into the cerebral spinal fluid, spreading through the spinal canal, where it's nearly impossible to remove surgically. I'd had this congenital brain tumor in-utero, which means that I was literally born with it. It's so rare, there are only around 100 cases a year,[1] and they're usually diagnosed in children under twelve. Lucky me.

And yet, I was so relieved to finally have a reason for what was wrong with me that when they told me there was a giant tumor in my head, I thought, *Thank God, it's something.* That "something," though, was about to upend my life.

I was told I might never play the piano again.

I'd trained for a decade to play professionally, and now it looked like I might lose the one thing that helped me define who I was as a person on this planet, in this universe. I was more afraid of not being able to be myself after cancer treatments career-wise, talent-wise, and passion-wise. If I couldn't play the piano, then who was I?

Nobody told us that the surgery itself had an 80 percent mortality rate. I'd find that out much later.

Step One: Surgery

Inside my waffle press of a mind, it was like, *Brain cancer? I'll just put some Windex on it, because I gotta get back to college to graduate. Doctors, can you just get this over with? I got a life to live, and this can't get in my way.*

I wasn't scared. Yet.

In the coming weeks, I'd endure the new patient Mad Hatter tea party: a flurry of doctors' visits, MRIs, pokes, prods, needles, scans, and *more* scans, not to mention the meds to reduce the swelling in my brain (my brain was swollen!), and the jerking off in a cup to a 27-inch Sony Trinitron TV with VCR tapes of porn, to preserve my sperm. It's a core trauma memory. (Did I mention infertility? Thanks, Mom, for driving me to the sperm bank! #awkward.)

As if all this medical indignity wasn't enough, there was the Storm of the Century that dropped several *feet* of snow in early January 1996, paralyzing New York City on the day of my surgery, pushing out the procedure till the next day, even though my dad was ready to dig out the car.

The surgery was a craniotomy, where they cut open your skull and have at it. It lasted for more than six-and-a-half hours. My neurosurgeon, who said the tumor popped out in three pieces like a matzah ball, reported, "I've never seen a tumor quite like this one, but I mean that in a good way." One of my doctors even called it "elegant," which I took to mean it looked good in pearls. I have no idea what he really meant, but he believed he'd managed to get clean margins, and that's all that mattered.

This was when I discovered there'd been only a 20 percent chance that I'd make it through the surgery in the first place because that tumor had been sitting on my spine. The medical staff obviously knew this because they insisted that I say goodbye to my parents before I was wheeled away. I watched Mom and Dad crying and hugging each other, their arms outstretched to me as I disappeared down the hallway.

When they visited me in the recovery room, I was so drugged up that I don't remember it. But my parents do. Dad wrote in his journal, "We were so emotional to see our son alive and well we cried for what felt like hours."

I'd survived brain surgery and yet, everything that had been normal and sacred in my life up to that moment, including my precious Jewfro, had come to a complete and abrupt end. One night, I was in the neurology ICU, recuperating from having my head cut open, my organs operated by machine for several hours, and enough anesthesia to take down a horse, when I heard the curtain pull back. Now, it's true that I was on high doses of morphine, but I know that there was an actual, honest-to-God priest standing there. He looked like the guy from *The Exorcist* sent to rid Linda Blair of demons.

Luckily, I'd been extubated, because before he could issue last rites or whatever Catholics do in the ICU, I "shouted" as best I could in a raspy voice, "I'm Jewish. I'm Jewish. I'm Jewish!" Miraculously, my semitic spell made him go away. I found out later he was there for the guy in the gurney next to me who didn't make it through the night. In hindsight, I could have used all the help I could have gotten.

The next morning, when I told my mom about my late-night visitor, she went all bat-shit Shirley MacLaine on the nursing staff, yelling, "You let a fucking priest talk to my fucking son after fucking brain surgery?"

Nobody warns you about these sorts of things. I guess because nobody expects them.

The day I got home from the hospital, I walked through the door and immediately sat down at the piano to play. I'd been playing some twenty times a day since I was eleven years old, but, throughout the fall and winter, my left hand was a limp nubbin lacking the fine motor skills to play right. Now I'd had surgery to remove a tumor from my head, and I was putting my fingers on the keys for the first time since.

I could play.

I could play.

I could play!

It wasn't as well as I used to, of course, because my muscles weren't quite working right. But I could play scales and that was enough to reunite with a piece of my soul, and I was so very happy.

Step Two: Radiation

After the surgery, I met with a radiation oncologist at a local hospital who was supposed to be in charge of the 33 radiation treatments I'd get to the head, neck, and spine. This is when my father stepped up to become the advocate for my health, asking, "How many college kids have you done this on for this exact condition?" The doctor replied, "None."

To quote Dr. Evil from *Austin Powers*, "How about no?"

We went to see Dr. Jeffrey Allen, a pediatric oncologist and quirky genius of a guy at what the hospital now called NYU Langone Health, who referred us to a radiation oncologist there. Only, I'd gained 80 pounds on Decadron, a steroid that shrinks tumors. That was even more weight than my future wife Jessica would later gain while pregnant with twins, and so, I was too big for the pediatric radiation tables. I was even too big for the adult radiation tables at that hospital, so I was sent uptown to Memorial Sloan Kettering Cancer Center.

First, I'd have to get fitted for a craniospinal mold for a cast that would immobilize me while they shot several lifetimes worth of radiation into my skull and spine. This was back before 3D imaging and precision robotics could create detailed maps of a patient's anatomy, back when they stuck us into form-fitting plastic casts. Some of them looked like cushy body-shaped beds, but mine looked like a cross between a mannequin's torso and Hannibal Lecter's mask.

The hardest part of the fitting was lying still for nearly four hours while they applied plaster of Paris to my entire body and added the netting for the mask to make a customized, full-body plastic "immobilization system." It was the most dehumanizing, demoralizing thing I've ever endured. I couldn't move, and I was in agony, drooling and crying. I begged for a break and something for the pain. I mean, I'd just had brain surgery and I was lying face down and completely still for the length of a Super Bowl broadcast. Maybe I could get an Ativan or a Percocet? Something? Compassion would have been nice.

Once the cast was ready, I came back for a trial treatment, minus the radiation, a sort of placebo zap to make sure the machine could maintain the right trajectory. On the way home, we stopped for lobster fra diavolo at Pier 17, which I then threw up somewhere along the Gowanus Expressway on the way to the bridge to Staten Island. I hurled dinner all over the sidewalk, nauseous even though they hadn't even turned on the lasers during the test treatment.

My father had to drive me to radiation every weekday because I couldn't drive myself, which, as far as I was concerned, was tragic. What twenty-something wants Daddy to drive him places? But I couldn't turn my head left or right. My mom was instrumental in helping me turn it millimeter by millimeter, tracking my improvement every day. When it came to my treatments and recovery, she'd otherwise retreated to the corners, unable to accept what was happening to her baby boy, but this she could handle.

Soon after I started weeks of radiation treatments, I began having some pretty horrible side effects: fatigue, nausea, and vomiting.

When I put it that way, it just sounds like a list rattled off at the end of a pharma commercial. No biggie. But it was way worse than it looks on paper, as in dry heaves that lasted twenty minutes causing muscle pain in my throat and stomach pain that lasted for days. There was "brain pain" that warranted codeine. Sometimes, I coughed up sputum all night, and I had diarrhea that waited for no man to get to the bathroom on time. I shit my pants three times en route to the toilet, and I threw up so often that I had a hard time keeping my meds down. It was actually news when, one night, I ate some pastina and it didn't come back up.

Soon, my throat swelled up and I could drink only Ensure or Boost. Well, that was before the ice cream diet was substituted in. I found it hard to swallow thin liquids because I would aspirate, so twice a day, my mom would bring home extra thick vanilla milkshakes from our neighborhood Carvel ice cream store. Eventually, she'd buy ten at a time, sticking them in the freezer.

I kept getting sicker and sicker while the radiation tried to make me healthier. Now I was scared. We begged my doctors for something to stop the vomiting and they gave me Kytril, an anti-emetic designed to mitigate chemo-induced nausea and vomiting. But it just reduced my vomiting from twenty times a day to five, and my mouth was perpetually dry at a time when the topline advice for managing loss of saliva was "chew gum." I found a tiny ad in one of the two cancer magazines available at the time touting a prescription medication for dry mouth. I ripped it out and brought it to my doctors, securing a prescription for eight pills at $50 a pop because, of course, they weren't covered by insurance. Worse, those magazines were filled with two types of ads: life insurance and reverse mortgages, as if to say, "You're gonna die. Might as well die wealthy."

I'll add that my parents joined me in the scared-shitless department, even though someone had to steer the ship as my primary caretaker. That someone was my dad. Not only did he chronicle every doctor's appointment, the names of every parking lot attendant, and every obstacle: *"SNOW, SNOW, SNOW!!!! 10 inches in*

Staten Island. I'm getting really fed up with snow!" He even recorded what and where I barfed:

> "*Matt gave up his dinner on 3rd Avenue and 39th Street. I cleaned his shoes, must demonstrate how to keep shoes clean when regurgitating.*"

My dad's obsessive accounting of every detail was his way of dealing with the fear of losing his son and maybe, to keep him from losing his shit. Maybe it was also an attempt to slow down and control time or otherwise contain the fallout from the meteor blast that had blown up our family life.

Every day, I slept about twenty-two hours and played the piano for an hour. It grounded me. I'd been writing symphonies for orchestras, jazz bands, and quintets, at school, but at home, all I had was one piano. So I started composing songs inspired by my medical savagery for what would eventually become a solo piano album called *Scribblings*.

But the radiation was taking its toll. My father begged my doctors to let me take a few days off so I could regain enough strength to withstand the side effects.

"He's going to die from this!" But they told us we had to finish the protocol, no deviations from the plan, which they'd made up anyway. I'm sure that if I'd skipped a day or two, I'd still be alive today.

As I finished up radiation, my doctors recommended chemotherapy, but they never explained to me what the side effects could be.

"Let's talk about chemo," they said.

"First, tell me when I'm going to die," I replied.

"Now that you've survived the surgery and radiation, we give you a 50 percent survival rate over the next five years." They sounded so certain, as though they'd plugged my info into a supercomputer and this got spit out. Medulloblastomas are frequently terminal, but I was three times the age of the average person who gets this diagnosis, and nobody really knew for sure.

"With the chemo, what does that bump the 50 percent up to?"
I added a bit of Gen X sass.

"Fifty-five percent, but we need to start immediately."

"I need time to think about it."

I called Uncle Jay. He called the hospital and, with our permission, got a hold of the chemo cocktail recipe. It was the usual suspects for medulloblastoma: cyclophosphamide, carboplatin, vincristine, and cisplatin, all blended into a concoction of toxic hell. It's what doctors call a "high-intensity regimen" that's used for aggressive cancers. Each has its job, mainly either killing cancer or keeping it from coming back.

Each also has its list of potential side effects, including nausea, vomiting, hair loss, low blood cell or platelet counts, increased risk of infection, fatigue, neuropathy, constipation, muscle weakness, hearing loss, nerve damage, and kidney toxicity. And that's just the short-term effects. Long-term effects can include chronic bladder conditions, infertility, kidney damage or failure, permanent hearing loss, and secondary cancers.

The chemo cocktail could also cause permanent nerve damage to my fingers and affect my hearing plus my cognitive function, all things you need for a career as a professional musician and film composer. Uncle Jay was concerned.

"Matt, I love you and I never thought I'd say these words to you," he said, "but you'd rather live a shorter life without these side effects than live longer with them. Don't let them take away your gift." He didn't want chemo to kill my career before it even got started. Neither did I, and so, I refused to take the chemo cocktail to boost my survival rate from 50 to 55 percent. When I told my doctors my decision, they were not happy.

"But we're trying to save your life."

I wasn't going to comply with the doctors simply because they said so, and I would rather take the risk of living a shorter life where I could play the piano, than a potentially longer one without it. Plus, I was sick of being poked and prodded and talked to like a child.

I finished my treatments, but I'd never really be done with cancer. None of us are. You can't go through something like that and return to your regularly scheduled life as though you hadn't just had your head cracked open, even in a controlled setting. Maybe that's the scariest part of it: cancer might leave your body, but it never leaves your life. I was forever changed by the diagnosis and the treatments, and not just because I later became a patient advocate. The entire ordeal took a toll on us all: the craniotomy and several dozen high-dose radiation treatments which, back then, were something like Chernobyl served through an Easy-Bake Oven. In all, I got about 3,000 lifetimes of our usual daily radiation exposure on Earth. Sadly, that's no exaggeration for comedic relief.

While my classmates were studying or partying, I was trying to adjust to cancer treatments. The most serious illness I should have been fighting was "senioritis" during my last semester of college. I'd instead taken on a tumor in my cerebellum, the part of the brain responsible for balance, judging distances, eye movements, speech, and our sense of timing. I gained 80 pounds from the steroids and then vomited out 110. I lost most of my muscle mass, my fertility, and all of my hair. And still, I had a 50 percent chance of making it to my twenty-sixth birthday.

Though doctors and nurses are among my favorite people—they saved my life, my brain, and my piano talent—the healthcare system isn't necessarily set up to support a patient's humanity. Not when the very first question they ask is, "What insurance do you have?"

While there are human moments among the institutional imbecility, there are also people like the doctor who explained the failure rate of post-cancer surgery, as my dad wrote, "coldly, as though Matt was a machine," throwing out words like "neurological decline" as nonchalantly as if he were predicting Saturday's weather. This, after his office had required us to pay for a fluoroscopy lumbar puncture, a spinal tap, up front: "*$618, Mastercard, of course.*"

Bottom line: Fear is an equal-opportunity employer. It afflicts patient and caregiver alike. And if you're a member of the sandwich generation, it afflicts you with triple idiocy: It's you, your parents, and your kids. It's also insidious because it gives you permission to stay stuck and feel hopeless. The alternative of leaning into hope means that you have to romance risk and find ways to keep on living, come what may, and that's no small task.

There Is No Spoon

Back when I was treated for cancer in the nineties, the healthcare system didn't offer much in the way of emotional support. There was no internet connecting like-minded cancer patients, and we were still very much in the "suck it up" phase of psychosocial culture. There was maybe a smattering of support groups and a pamphlet or two about what to expect when you have cancer, but none of what they said to expect was what I got.

Case in point: I was given postcards that listed potential side effects that, I was assured, were "unlikely," and I was supposed to fill in the boxes on the off chance that I experienced any of them. Then they would deal with anything that might come up, even though that was (checks notes) "unlikely."

Yet each time I went back for treatments, I'd hand them a post-card with every single box checked off in smelly black marker. They behaved as though they'd never seen this before, pinning me as the problem patient. I didn't fit into a box, even though I'd checked all of them off.

To me, it was all a horrible, no-good nuisance to get through so I could get back to playing the piano and graduating from college. I wasn't offered much of it outside of my inner circle of family and friends and maybe I wouldn't have accepted it anyway. I'd like to think I was just being Zen, like the message from the "There is no spoon" scene from *The Matrix*. It's when an (impossibly young) Keanu Reeves is in the waiting room to see the Oracle to determine if he's "The One," and he watches a bald kid dressed like a Buddhist monk bend a spoon with his mind. The boy tells him, "Do not try and bend the spoon. That's impossible. Instead, only try to realize the truth . . . there is no spoon. Then you'll see that it is not the spoon that bends; it is only yourself."

In other words, logic is futile. And if there's one thing cancer patients can understand it's that logic only gets you so far, and overcoming fear is a Herculean effort that I'm not sure is entirely helpful. You see it in the military terms that people use when it comes to the "war on cancer." You're labeled a "fighter," tossed into the Thunderdome of the "slash/burn/poison" of surgery/radiation/chemo to "battle the enemy."

But I do not believe that people who die of cancer didn't fight hard enough. They probably just got shitty odds from a terrible cancer or subpar treatments barely paid for by crappy insurance. Or maybe they got all of the above.

Meanwhile, they're bombarded by cheerful sayings in their Instagram feed, offering books with titles like, *Feel the Fear and Do it Anyway* or GIFs of the Winston Churchill quote, "If you're going through hell, keep going." When you do just that, everyone praises you for your strength, when really, you're just doing the shit you have to because, what are your choices?

In the three decades since I had a tumor squatting on my cerebellum, I learned that when you're a cancer patient, it's the best time ever to give yourself some grace. Cancer is scary, and it's okay to feel terrified. No one prepares for this type of fear unless you are a hypochondriac, and I'm not sure that all that anxious training prepares anyone for the real thing. It's the people born with congenital moxie who tend to fare better.

So cut yourself some slack, because it's simply human instinct to fight or flight, and flight doesn't necessarily have to be option B. These reactions are evolutionary biology, developed across millions of years, so that we have the ability to react and respond ideally in a way that benefits us when danger appears.

People say fear is a choice. I think that's a very weirdly user-defined, dogmatic, existential way to think about it. Sometimes you need fear because it helps guide you and protect you. Maybe you want to cocoon off into the bathroom and cry, or you want to start journaling your story. Or maybe you're the type who faces fear by showing up for a cancer walk in a Superman cape, letting your freshly bald head shine and your freak flag fly. There are no wrong answers here.

No matter what you choose for your own self-preservation, understand that fear is okay. Give yourself permission to be afraid because there's really nothing wrong with it. There's nothing wrong with *you*.

The fear of death and mortality is very real, but if you're a pragmatist, you may understand that we're all a day away from death every day anyhow. Maybe you're paralyzed by fear one day and sporting a "My oncologist does my hair" T-shirt the next. You're allowed the ups and downs.

Here's the hard truth: Life is not fair. Without good, there's no evil, and without evil, there's no good. There has to be bad shit, and that's terrible, especially when you're standing in it. But if everything was always rosy and happy, that wouldn't be living. That'd be an episode of *Caillou*.

I'm a big fan of trying to figure out how to surrender to the current instead of fighting it. That's how they tell you to get out of a rip current, a dangerous rogue channel of water that has felled many a swimmer. The people who fight it don't always make it back to shore. Here's what you're supposed to do instead:

1. Stay calm.
2. Conserve your energy by floating.
3. Swim parallel to the shore, no matter how badly you want to try to swim right at it.
4. Signal for help.

Of course, I could just as easily come up with a metaphor where fighting is the correct solution to the problem, perhaps something with ninjas or the subway. Fight or flight, you do you, and your cancer treatments will do what they do. But please, give yourself grace no matter what you choose on any given day, and when you need it, signal for help.

I guess what I'm trying to say is, there really is no spoon.

When You're Still Deep in It (Also, Afterward)

When you're on day one and day two and day three and day four of this nightmare you've found yourself in, it's hard to find your way. Nowadays, though, there are directories in this store that you never wanted to shop in. In this century, we have emotional support services for cancer patients and their caregivers, and it's generally thought of as acceptable to need it and to get it. That's relatively new.

I can't stress enough how important it is from the perspective of history, progress, society, empathy, and community that these days, we give a shit about your well-being, and not just your biology. We care not only that cancer patients live, but *how* they live after or with cancer, if you've got the kind that sticks around.

It took a while for us all to get here. For a long time, society simply wasn't ready to think beyond the physical when it came to illness.

English speakers put the words "psycho" and "social" together way back in 1891 to create the word "psychosocial," meaning, "pertaining to or involving the influence of social factors on a person's mind or behavior."[2] In other words, life affects your mood. Who knew?

This was the Sigmund Freud-Carl Jung era of psychology, when we started looking at how other things, people, situations, and penis envy affected our behavior. It was also when many illnesses were attributed to moral failings and cancer was discussed in hushed tones. So, it was a slow start.

It would be another century before the word started appearing in our vernacular more frequently, and I was raised during the upswing, though it was more of a sloth-climbing-a-tree than a swing (Figure 3.1). There's a reason we Gen Xers sometimes behave like

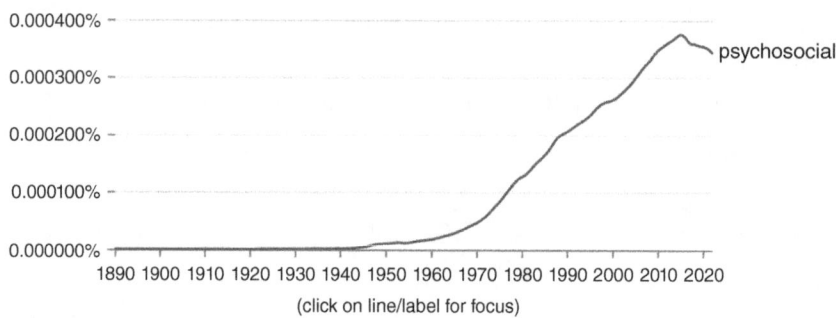

FIGURE 3.1 Trends of Psychosocial.
Source: Google Ngram Viewer (*Psychosocial—Etymology, Origin & Meaning*)

a pack of feral dogs. We were the generation that drank from hoses because we weren't allowed inside the house all day. If we complained about it—or anything—we'd hear, "I'll give you something to cry about."

Cancer will give you a good cry, that's for sure, and yet even in 1996, people weren't exactly encouraged to feel feelings and surely not to show them. There just weren't many resources to give cancer patients some emotional guidance, no handrails, no sherpas, no nothing.

Now, though? There's a shit-ton, maybe too much. But being aware that there are patient support groups, not to mention cutesy hand-painted signs and clever T-shirts, and all sorts of infrastructure to help you through it is a nice thing to have.

Remember, in Freud's time, cancer was pretty much a death sentence, and hospitals were a place to go and die. The word "anesthesiologist" wasn't coined until 1902,[3] and the FDA didn't approve its first chemotherapy drug until decades later, in 1949. That drug was mechlorethamine, a derivative of mustard gas, which was used in chemical warfare during World War II. After Germans dropped it on American warships in Italy, doctors observed that the chemical lowered white blood cell counts. Somebody then hypothesized that it could keep cancer cells from dividing and voila! Chemo was born.[4]

For the longest time, there wasn't support for cancer survivors because there weren't many of them. Back 125 years ago, doctors were feared and curative treatments were few and far between. Thanks to cancer research and advances in oncology (and BTW, bedside manner), overall[i] cancer five-year survival rates went from 38 percent[5] in the late 1960s to nearly 70 percent[6] today. Some cancers, like Hodgkin's lymphoma and thyroid cancer, have five-year survival rates in the ninetieth percentile.

There are an estimated 26 million predicted to walk among us by 2040[7] and I hope I'm one of them, perhaps shouting at my personal robot to bring me a bowl of ice cream and my drone footage of the last known polar bear. Meanwhile, I want to make healthcare suck less, and that includes the psychosocial part.

The truth is, I lost my life but I didn't die. I took to the couch while my friends, all in their twenties and having the time of their lives, were off to new jobs or graduate school. There was no Facebook page or Instagrammed photos of the stitches in my head to remind them of what I was going through, and nobody was about to drive three hours to Staten Island to watch me throw up.

I managed to return to school, against doctor's orders, and graduated on time, earning a BA with honors in Music and Computers and a final GPA of 3.7—magna cum laude, thank you very much. But I wasn't the same Matt.

I had to retrain the muscles in my hand to play the piano again. I didn't go to grad school. Instead, I got a job changing ink cartridges in computer printers and later, fixing computers in an advertising agency. Plan B became Plan A.

Cancer survivorship wasn't yet a thing, and it surely wasn't on the radar for someone barely old enough to legally order a beer at a New York Rangers game. I was supposed to be happy to be alive— and I was. But I wasn't supposed to want a "normal life," whatever the

---

[i]Includes all types of cancer and people of all ages combined. Your mileage may vary.

hell that was. Jobs, spouse, kids? A 30-year mortgage and life insurance? Not getting the taste of MRI scan contrast in my mouth whenever an interviewer asked, "Where do you see yourself in five years?"

But I wasn't the only young adult cancer survivor, or the only medulloblastoma survivor, or the only survivor in New York, or the only person to ever have brain surgery. My people, like your people, are out there. It's a matter of finding them and connecting with them, because if there's anyone who understands the brand of fear you've faced and the kind of support you need, it's someone like you. It's We the Survivors.

4   We the Purpose-Seekers

I didn't mean to piss off Hollywood, but to be fair, they pissed me off first. I wrote about it in a 2007 rant in *The Huffington Post*, since wiped from the internet, called, "Stand Down to Cancer, Another Waste of Time." In it, I took issue with the impending launch of the celebrity-laden, Hollywood-backed advocacy group Stand Up to Cancer. I was adamant that the last thing that the cancer community needed was yet another appeal for money, shot in stark black-and-white video with tinkling piano keys and violins setting the somber mood for the poor, poor little cancer patients. I predicted it would bring nothing more than stunts in the name of cancer, like shaving off your hair for the cure, and "pinkwashing" kind of bullshit where brands co-opt the cause to sell carcinogenic stuff in pretty colors. Here was Hollywood showing up yet again with an empty promise to cure cancer and make life better for our beloved headscarved. No, thank you.

I thought that maybe a handful of people would read my guest post, hopefully some fellow young adult cancer survivors with a penchant for snark. Suddenly, my cell phone rang. This was back in the day when we were still mostly using landlines and your cell was reserved for emergencies, so I was surprised and a little alarmed.

"Hello?"

A voice said, "Please hold for Laura Ziskin."

Ziskin was a powerhouse Hollywood producer. I'm talking, *Pretty Woman* and the Spider-Man franchise. She was also a co-founder of Stand Up to Cancer, and she had a plan to turn the pain of her own breast cancer story into a research-based mission for early detection of all cancers with a goal of reducing cancer deaths by 50 percent within a decade. But in the months before the launch, it looked to me like her organization was doing nothing more than planning yet another bald-patient pity party.

With just 750 words on Arianna Huffington's online newspaper, I'd managed to shit on not only Stand Up to Cancer's mission, but on its nine co-founders, including Paramount Pictures CEO Sherry Lansing and America's sweetheart Katie Couric. When Ziskin came to the phone, she barked, "I don't know who you are and I don't like what you wrote, but I need to know you."

After our brief call, I contacted Dr. Leonard Sender, a rock star of an adolescent and young adult (AYA) oncologist, who would become the chairman of my nonprofit.

"Lennie, we've been summoned by Laura Ziskin to meet her at Sony Studios. I think I pissed her off."

We met up in her Hollywood office with twenty-five-foot ceilings and posters of famous movies like *Men in Black* and *Rain Man* on the walls. It looked like the set of an Orson Welles movie, and it felt like that moment in *The Wizard of Oz* when the screen goes from boring black and white to magical full Technicolor. I was so intimidated, I nearly shit my pants. I wondered: *Why the fuck am I here?* With that, Laura Ziskin marched into the room, pointed at me, and said, "Do you have any idea how hard it is to get the nine most powerful women in Hollywood to agree on *anything*?"

We became instant friends. She wanted to know who was this angry kid, young enough to be her son, and whether I might throw another wrench into her plans. I was able to convince her that she couldn't pull off her fledgling organization's mission without buy-in from the

AYA cancer community. Generation X had to be their advocates or else they'd come across as nothing more than Hollywood hubris.

The way cancer research had always worked was like sprinkling kibble out for scientists to gobble up as they scampered from laboratory to laboratory for funding. But what Ziskin's Hollywood heavyweights wanted to do instead was convene doctors and scientists to find research that needed funding. It was antithetical to the agendas of research and fundraising hubs like Johns Hopkins Medicine and the American Cancer Society. It was, instead, a dream team chasing science, not money. Bring the younger generation along, I told Ziskin, putting patients on advisory boards to tell real-life stories.

The truth is, we were on the same side, both of us survivors trying to make cancer suck less. She was a Hollywood hotshot, and though I'd started making a name for myself, I certainly wasn't Sony Pictures C-suite-level famous. Yet, I was fast becoming the Forrest Gump of cancer advocacy, always winding up in the right place with the right people at the right time. Sometimes, they'd even summon me.

It was the year I launched I'm Too Young for This! (i[2]y), an AYA cancer advocacy organization, from my spare bedroom in Brooklyn, which I called, "Headquarters," the homebase of what would one day become the world's largest AYA cancer advocacy organization.

We were becoming a movement of young, ticked off largely Gen X cancer survivors who wanted their voices heard, and that was notably new. Until then, cancer advocacy was largely pediatric or geriatric. Or pink ribbons. And it was killing us.

The stark data was laid out in a 2006 report[1] by heavy governmental hitters, including the US Department of Health and Human Services, the National Institutes of Health, and the National Cancer Institute, in conjunction with LIVESTRONG's Young Adult Alliance: ". . . compared with younger and older age groups, this population—defined as those diagnosed with cancer at ages 15 through 39—has seen little or no improvement in cancer survival rates for decades."

Back then, as now, the average cancer patient was old enough to receive Medicare. Meanwhile, pediatric cancer patients made up just

0.75 percent of all cancers and yet, says *CancerScope*, children's cancer has "had enormous research, training, and clinical care directed toward them."[2] They're also way cuter than the rest of us, which is why you see photos of bald kids and not thirty-year-old project managers on those "leave a quarter" fundraising boards at deli checkout counters.

Meanwhile, nobody was addressing what it was like to get a cancer diagnosis between final exams, or while dating, or while starting a career or a family, all things that generally didn't affect eighty-year-olds. We were mad as hell, and we weren't going to take it anymore. *I* wasn't going to take it anymore.

I had been forever scarred by the lack of humanity I experienced during my cancer treatments, and I didn't want anyone else to feel the way I had: like nobody cared about anything but getting the cancer out. Back in the nineties, the radiation rooms I spent a total of nearly fifty hours in were built like bank vaults with thick doors to protect everyone outside from dangerous radiation. We patients were led into the vault and abandoned, left to smell the cancerous laser shit that radiates your body like you're Three Mile Island in a cotton hospital gown.

I desperately longed for something that would help soothe my nerves during the ninety-minute treatments, so I asked if I could listen to my music during the zapping. Music had long been my refuge and my reason for living, and I needed something to get me through this radioactive hell. I was told a big, fat, "No, we don't do that."

So one day, I showed up with my double cassette tape portable music player and some songs I'd recorded in college and announced, "I'm listening to this." No headphones. Just an old school silver boombox like the one John Cusack held over his head to blast "In Your Eyes" in *Say Anything*. I demanded my music for my own personal well-being so that I didn't have to suffer through another hour-and-a-half of boring and terrifying radiation, feeling like I was dying alone. They relented, and for the first time ever, there was music inside the radioactive vaults at Sloan Kettering. That boombox is probably radiating a landfill somewhere.

This was the spirit of i[2]y, making a stand for our very souls and for our youth. But I wouldn't have launched it without some encouragement by some important people. If anyone accelerated me into this cancer advocacy rabbit hole in the first place, it was my doppelgänger, Craig Lustig, a bald, Jewish, New York City-based, twentysomething brain tumor survivor who had been in the a cappella group I work with at SUNY Binghamton, though we didn't know each other then. We became friends after he saw me perform before thousands of people on the National Mall for the American Cancer Society's Celebration on the Hill.

"You should be a cancer advocate," he said, to which I replied, "The fuck is a cancer advocate?"

Craig was serving on the board of the National Coalition of Cancer Survivors (NCCS), and he knew all the cancer advocacy insiders and he thought I had what it took to join them.

"You'd make life suck less for the next twenty-one-year-old brain tumor patient." He wanted me to make sure that the next college kid who gets cancer isn't given Robitussin and sent home.

"I'm in," I said. "What do I do?"

I jumped right in. On the i[2]y YouTube channel, I posted a few public service announcements that I'd recorded with a presmartphone, low-res webcam. I was very proud when the channel racked up a thousand views in the first week, a testament to the success of the Bob Dylan–style flashcard videos shot in front of a hanging bedsheet. Here are a few samples:

1. "1 in 10 cancer survivors is under 40."
2. "There are over 10 million cancer survivors in the U.S."[i]
3. "That's over one million survivors under 40!!!"

That same year, *TIME* magazine deemed the i[2]y website among its top 50 of the year, which was hilarious, because the site was

---

[i]Now it's 19 million.

basically a hand-coded, cobbled-together aggregate portal of AYA cancer resources and a calendar of local gatherings around the country. Ranked seventeenth on *TIME's* list, it somehow even beat LinkedIn and Yelp.

The New York Times quoted me in a round-up about AYA cancer, I was also quoted in *The Wall Street Journal* and *Newsday*, and *The Washington Post* called it "an unparalleled resource for cancer patients in their teens, twenties, and thirties."[3]

Meanwhile, I launched the *Stupid Cancer Show*, an internet talk livestream, or, for the kids, what we now call a "podcast" only you had to tune in at a certain time like it was *The Love Boat* circa 1978. In time, I'd be dubbed the "Podfather of Healthcare," calling out healthcare goonery with "a mic in one hand and a middle finger on the other."

We promoted everyone, welcoming all sorts of organizations, from health brands to pharma firms, biotech to insurance companies, and we featured survivors and advocates. It was real talk for real people, addressing the psychosocial issues that AYA survivors face, such as cancer and pregnancy, survivorship, working while sick, sexuality, the cannabis debate, and cancer types that tend to affect younger adults like melanoma, Hodgkin's lymphoma, and testicular cancer.

Eventually, I moved the show's HQ from our spare bedroom to an abandoned, cemented elevator shaft in a city building in Tribeca. So, here's Cancer Kid, shoved into a windowless room without HVAC until we had enough money to move into a real office with windows and desks and doors that open and close.

Within five years, we reached half-a-million listeners. Eventually, we racked up 4.5 million listens. I'd become the Howard Stern of cancer, and I'd found purpose in the very bad thing that had happened to me. I created the support I wished I'd had when I was a cancer patient on the radiation table listening to the vault door close, leaving me with my fears and loneliness.

Meanwhile, Margaret Nagel, an Emmy-winning Hollywood producer, told me about a new show she was working on for Lifetime that was like *Ally McBeal*, but in an ad agency—if Ally had brain cancer. Margaret asked for my help to make the cancer storyline authentic. She had seen photos of our inaugural Stupid Cancer Happy Hour in Washington, DC on Myspace, and she wanted me to write a scene for her show. So, I did.

I put the lead character into one of our happy hours, packing the scene with the raw, unfiltered reality of what it's like to be a young adult with cancer. There were jokes, tears, awkward silences, and "cancertinis," and I was proud of it. I hit Send.

Margaret sent me the scene back with a notable edit: she'd added a character named Matthew, who would be the emcee of the happy hour, and declared, "You're going to play yourself."

I soon found myself on the set of *Side Order of Life* in exotic Pasadena, welcoming the show's main characters into the "club no one wants to belong to" and wondering how the hell my life had turned into a literal Lifetime movie. Oh, and Jason Priestley was on set. Gen X women, swoon!

It was the first time AYA cancer was given a national platform in the mainstream American pop culture zeitgeist. Yes, we had LIVESTRONG back then, and I somehow became tapped for a small part of their mission, the Young Adult Alliance. Though the yellow wristband cancer organization wasn't 100 percent AYA-specific, i[2]y was, and it was growing fast.

Two years into the venture, I made my first hire, Kenny Kane, a kid from Islip, Long Island, who was finishing up his final year of college and needed a ninety-hour internship to graduate. He'd heard about i[2]y during a presentation by the head of our Long Island chapter.

"I knew that everybody in the room was probably perked up for an internship," Kenny remembered. "So I actually got in trouble for emailing Matt during this woman's presentation because I wanted to be the first one in for an internship request." When he graduated, he became i[2]y's second full-time employee.

Kenny's father had survived testicular cancer at age fifty, heading from chemo straight to Kenny's high school graduation. Though

Kenny wasn't a survivor, he was survivor-adjacent, and together, we were the perfect duo. Somebody called him the Spuds McKenzie of AYA cancer, and that fits. Spuds was the super cool bull terrier mascot in Bud Light commercials back when Gen X was in college. Kenny was cool and he was loyal.

But to me, Kenny was my Jack Skellington, the master of ceremonies, the "Pumpkin King" from *The Nightmare Before Christmas*, who kept the show running for years. He built our e-commerce site, and he's the mastermind behind our first wristbands, black i[2]y "Give Cancer the Bird" bands that smelled at first like, well, cancer, from the off-gassing of nasty ingredients like formaldehyde. The "bird" in question was the kind you'd see a New York cabbie throw at you when you cut him off, but we also offered a kid-friendly version that wouldn't get anyone sent to the principal's office. It helped that *High School Musical* actor Zac Efron took to wearing them to support the cause, lending his celebrity as our spokesperson.

"It was really a marketing vehicle that we made a little bit of profit on," Kenny told me, estimating that merch sales by 2016 were about $275,000 a year.

By 2012, I knew we'd made AYA cancer advocacy a legitimate movement when, now rebranded as Stupid Cancer after my internet radio show of the same name, we took 650 Gen X cancer survivors to the Palms Casino in Las Vegas for the three-day OMG! Cancer Summit for Young Adults, the predecessor of CancerCon.

This event would never pass today's quick-to-cancel standards. We'd plopped cancer survivors into a casino with cigarette smoke, gambling, booze, Playboy bunnies, and a rooftop pool in the direct desert melanoma-producing sun. But it was exactly what we needed.

We had an in through our chairman, Dr. Leonard "Lennie" Sender, who knew billionaire Palms owner George Maloof. Then Volkswagen donated a Beetle Turbo for the *Get Busy Living* tour, named after my favorite line from *Shawshank Redemption*. Kenny drove it from New York to Las Vegas, stopping in ten cities for events made for young adult cancer survivors and their caregivers. At the conference, we did a skit where we pretended I was in the trunk the whole time.

People shared their cancer journeys and the most AYA cancer story won the Get Busy Living Award and a two-year loan of a 2012 Passat TDI. It was an *American Idol*–style giveaway, with the finalists on stage and the grand prize going to whoever had the saddest cancer story.

That weekend, we featured comedians, jugglers, workshops, plenaries, social events, and a keynote by Will Reiser, the young guy who wrote the screenplay for the semi-autobiographical AYA cancer movie *50/50*, which we screened. I told an interviewer, "What we're doing has never been done before, and that's why it's an extraordinary moment in history."[4]

It was the year it all began to make sense, all the work, all the effort, all the hustle. It was the year that it all began to matter. I'd set out to build a movement, not an organization, and it was clear we'd succeeded. We finally had some real data that our community was contributing to Institutional Review Board (IRB) studies, research that involves humans to measure the effects of diagnoses and treatments on certain populations. We could throw up a survey on our Facebook page on a Friday and by Sunday, we'd have quality data on oncofertility or the psychological effects of cancer treatments on young adults. Stupid Cancer started to show up in the references on slides at oncology association meetings, and soon, AYA cancer research became a protocol, not just a "nice to have." Over the years, our community has contributed to cancer research on survivorship, caregiving, parenting, sexuality, disability, identity, financial toxicity, social media, genetic counseling, pain, anxiety, and much more.

"We created stickiness," Kenny said. "We were like the MTV of cancer," because musicians all went on MTV back in the day. If you were in AYA cancer, you came on our radio show, just like Dire Straits and Madonna were on MTV in its earliest days. "We were the shit," Kenny said.

That fall, I was invited to attend the Stand Up to Cancer telethon, and I met with "50/50's" Will Reiser and actor Seth Rogen, thanking them for what they've done for the cause. Like I said, I'm Forrest Gump. I never set out to be a cancer advocate/mouthpiece/champion/rabble-rouser but that's exactly where I ended up.

Until then, I just wanted to be able to play the piano again and to eventually return to my old life, whatever that meant. But when I hit the so-called "re-entry" stage after treatments ended, I found that survivorship programs for young adults were few and far between. The oncology landscape was analog and isolating, and only a handful of upstart AYA rapscallions were talking about our unique needs, our challenges, and our voices.

Yet I was born not just with a brain tumor, but with an inherent disdain for authority. When authority was suddenly in charge of whether or not I'd live and how it all affected me psychosocially, I was pissed off enough to do something about it. I related to Don Music, the piano-playing Muppet who would bang his head on his keys in frustration when things didn't go his way. Don was cancelled from the show in the nineties after parents reportedly complained that their kids were imitating his self-inflicted head-banging, but I always had a soft spot in my heart for him. I understood how he felt, and never more so than when I got cancer.

Please understand that I'm grateful for the access to the best treatments of the times, and I know I'm privileged in many ways. But I came out of the entire cancer ordeal angry at how I was treated—like a piece of biology, not a person. There were plenty of other people who felt the same way, and i[2]y let us bang our heads on our keyboards, so to speak. Until then, nearly every cancer organization had been built by academics, social scientists, health economists, researchers, and oncology professionals, with some celebrities thrown into the mix. What was missing was righteous anger that only comes from the people who'd endured it all.

If You Build It

Stupid Cancer wasn't built by a committee but by our community, and that was important to me. From our humble beginnings of just one person in a spare bedroom with no board, no money, no nothing, it was, at first, just me and my idea. I knew I couldn't do what I wanted to if I formed an LLC or an S Corp; it had to be a nonprofit, a 501(c)(3). The only thing is, I knew nothing about running a nonprofit, and I had no right to even try.

I'd learned a bit about branding while working as tech support for advertising agencies. I serviced Macintosh computers, which meant that I worked with creatives, and through them, I learned about all things desktop publishing, including software like Adobe and Quark, and design principles, like kerning and fonts. I wound up living and breathing in the creative space, fixing computers for a boutique ad agency.

This background gave me an appreciation for LIVESTRONG's sleek yellow-and-black branding. It wasn't the usual pink ribbons and heart-tugging patient photos. I mean, LIVESTRONG used a modern, clean, and friendly sans serif font, and their yellow was always consistent across all their marketing materials. I could see it even though I'm color blind! Their branding would even hold up today, if it wasn't for the eventual cancellation of Lance Armstrong for doping while cycling a few years later. For us, however, LIVES-TRONG was like a machete hacking through the forest to make a dirt road. Thanks to them, we could come along and make the highway.

A series of mentors led the way for me, starting with Ellen Stovall. A Stage IV Hodgkin's lymphoma survivor at twenty-four, she went on to pioneer cancer survivorship as the President and CEO of the National Coalition for Cancer Survivorship (NCCS), the oldest survivor-led advocacy organization, now called Cancer Nation. (See Chapter 5.) She said that quality of life should be tantamount to quality of care. (That shouldn't have been revolutionary, but it was.) She helped me understand cancer advocacy and showed me how to structure my organization.

Carol Cone, the "mother of cause marketing," a sort of female Don Draper of the late twentieth century, was another influence. When the CEO at the agency where I worked introduced me to her, Carol helped me appreciate Stupid Cancer's brand promise, which was far from the usual Hallmark "get well" card feel of most cancer organizations. Instead of a cancer pity party, we gave AYA cancer survivors permission to be pissed off and offered an outlet to do something about it with like-minded people.

Together, these two women triggered the Pygmalion effect on me, where I performed better because they expected me to, crafting my niche market and monetizing without being donor-dependent, all for the cause. We were fighting to be seen for who we were, not just what we had, and Stupid Cancer became a cohesive place for AYA survivors to gather together and share the unshareable, the things that might scare off family and friends, with other people in the trenches. It was a release valve, a much-needed collective scream. Just like in *Field of Dreams*, we built it, and they came, and I swear that FOMO fueled us, the MTV of AYA cancer, for the first few years. People asked:

"Can we have a meetup?"
"Can I come to the conference?"
"Can we be listed on your website?"
"Can I come on your radio show?"

We were the first in this space, and people were clamoring to be a part of it. I guess we looked bigger than we were, but in the beginning, this "we" was really just me. My wife, Jessica, and I didn't have kids yet, and so I had the time and the drive to build and to build fast, and Jessica didn't mind. I appreciated her patience and her corporate-sponsored health insurance. With the help of a handful of intrepid volunteers, I handled the branding, the graphics, the coding, the design, and the printing.

Kenny was such an integral part of my humble beginnings that it's hard to overstate how important he was to our growth. We lived and breathed i[2]y, and we even lived in the same building when my kids were babies, and we commuted to work together every day.

Alli Ward came on board in 2011 to run our OMG! Cancer Summit for Young Adults, and she did it for free. I didn't have the money to pay her, and anyhow, she said, "Sure, why not. I've got nothing to lose. I'm dying anyway."[5] Alli had been diagnosed in 2009 with stage IV ovarian cancer, which was discovered after a surgeon opened her abdomen up to remove an ovarian cyst before it could burst. The cancer had spread to her liver, so she had surgery, chemo, and radiation, but nothing was working. She stopped treatments to concentrate on her quality of life during what was expected to be just months left of living. She'd been told to get her affairs in order, so she'd quit her job, sold her house, and moved in with her parents.

Two years later, she was, in fact, still living, past her "expiration date," as she put it. So why not organize a conference for hundreds of young adult cancer patients? She'd serve as our vice president of programs and development through 2015, and later, as Chief Operating Officer. In 2018, she spoke at our annual CancerCon, sharing the story of the living miracle that she is.

"Though I did not die, cancer had taken over my life. I could barely see the person I was before cancer . . . all the things that I felt identified me and made me happy were absent from my life." She told us a story about how she'd quit hiking, believing the voice in her head that told her she was no longer strong enough. But then she went on a hiking trip to Alaska with her husband and stepdaughters anyhow, and, she said while sharing a photo from the trip, "I am on the top of that fucking mountain." The audience roared. "Sorry, Matt, I swore." The voice in her head had been wrong. "I'm going to live and love my life to the fullest."[6]

From the beginning, Lennie played the role of our angry Boomer, a doctor without a single ounce of imposter syndrome. (I had enough of it for us all.) A hematology oncologist at Children's Hospital of Orange County, he'd been treating adolescents and young adults since I was in third grade. He was our chairman and my big brother, my staunchest defender, an incomparable and unassailable leader, and my dearest BFF and partner in crime. Without him, Stupid Cancer would not have happened at all.

Lennie understood firsthand that AYA cancer was woefully behind other age groups in terms of research and resources, not to mention attention. He worked with us to write an Adolescent and Young Adult Cancer Bill of Rights, which was endorsed by more than two dozen organizations, including the mighty Leukemia & Lymphoma Society, now called Blood Cancer United, the owner of many of those "leave a quarter" boards. Among the rights are to:

- be listened to and heard when seeking a diagnosis and discussing treatment options.
- feel comfortable and trusted in your care. There is nothing wrong with switching doctors.
- have open conversations early in your treatment planning about the impact of your treatment on future fertility and a discussion about your fertility preservation options.
- understand the financial impact of cancer treatment and receive information and support to help plan accordingly.
- receive information about clinical trials that may be beneficial to your treatment and survivorship.
- look forward to a productive future.[7]

Together with other organizations, we developed a groundbreaking movement for a long-ignored segment of cancer patients with unique issues, such as post-treatment fertility. We took on questions like, should you stay in school? Go on dates? How can we afford treatments if we can't keep working? Should we move back in with our parents? As I told *The Wall Street Journal* in 2010, "We give angry young adult survivors a home."[8]

The Media Machine

To build our network, we took advantage of social media, which was brand-spanking new, and blogging, which was king. Though we had 50,000 followers on Myspace, people would ask, "What's Myspace?" We had work to do.

Back then, it was a novel superpower to be able to organize so easily and quickly. There were no influencers, no "click like and follow for more," no waking up to tens of thousands of new followers because a post went viral. The biggest cancer organizations were still mailing out flyers and processing actual paper checks.

But young nurses and doctors in their twenties and thirties saw us online and embraced us for the angry digital mob we were, and the legacy media was already taking note. We were among the first nonprofits to have a Facebook page, the first to do e-commerce. The first with merch, and that merch funded a lot of what we did.

We had some role models from the dial-up days of AOL (America Online), back when people had to hope that no one in the house would pick up the phone and knock them off the internet. I tip my hat to AOL's AIDS forums of the nineties and the first cancer forum, for testicular cancer, founded by my buddy Steve Friedman back before Lance Armstrong was even diagnosed. They leveraged the burgeoning technology to build community where it had been lacking.

Not that it was easy even in the 2000s, when Facebook was still a dot-edu website, YouTube and Twitter were brand new, and Instagram and TikTok didn't yet exist. I hand-coded our newsletters and turned them into PDFs using some weird, crappy Adobe hack I'd figured out.

I told the editors of a 2008 California HealthCare Foundation report that I believed the cancer "establishment" of the time had not been supporting us, so I created an open-source aggregate of resources that would.[9] Our website featured a social events calendar for happy hours in places like DC, Boston, and Ontario. We linked to sites like Lotsa Helping Hands and CarePages, and we offered forums, chatrooms, and bulletin boards where AYA survivors could share and support one another. We included links to forums for ovarian cancer, colon cancer, testicular cancer, and lymphoma, and of course, we sold irreverent merch.

That was very important to us, because we'd seen the success of LIVESTRONG's wristband sales. They cost just 15 cents to make and sold for a dollar each. By 2005, the yellow bands were appearing on the wrists of celebrities and entire sports teams. By the 2010s, LIVESTRONG, with the help of Nike's branding experts, had sold more than $100 million worth of them. In the 2000s, LIVESTRONG was a formidable marketing machine.

Our black wristband with the middle finger was our first item in the store, and by 2012, we were selling out $20 T-shirts that said simply, "Stupid Cancer." As Kenny wrote, "People didn't just want to donate; they wanted to *wear* their support. They wanted to make a statement."[10] In the beginning, we used Cafe Press' print-on-demand fulfillment services, so no one had a basement full of swag. Besides, we were a nonprofit, so our donor dollars couldn't fund merch.

Kenny scaled our store and as we grew, our product line expanded to offer more colors, more sizes, more items. A third party took care of fulfillment. It was, as Kenny wrote, a "visibility engine," not really a fundraiser. "Every person wearing a Stupid Cancer shirt was a walking billboard for the movement."[11]

We've since fulfilled thousands of orders all while building our brand literally on Gen X's—and now, Millennials' and Generation Z's—backs. Not everyone understood what we were doing, of course. Plenty of times people would stop me on the street, point at my T-shirt, and ask, "Why is cancer stupid?" I would just say, "You're right. Cancer is not stupid. It's a really smart disease." Then I'd walk away, because it wasn't worth explaining to people who didn't immediately get it deep in their radiated bones. But our people totally understood.

It wasn't just us "kids" behind this movement. Our medical advisory council included some pretty big names in medicine, including Bernie Siegel, MD, author of the seminal *Love, Medicine & Miracles*, MD, and Andrew Weil, MD, not to mention my own neuro-oncologist, Dr. Allen. This helped legitimize us among the medical community, which tends to keep patients in a separate bucket.

After just a few years, Fox News named i[2]y one of the best health blogs,[12] citing our goal of helping "patients help themselves so they can continue to live their lives." We kept up our support by offering copies of cancer survivorship publications, listed under the heading, "Advocacypalooza." We shared information about cancer-specific escapes through survivor retreats on ranches and outdoor experiences in the Rockies. Most of all, we gave people the right to be angry at how healthcare treats us.

We explained: "It takes more than 'being cured' to survive cancer. (What does 'cured' mean anyway?) It takes resilience, creativity, audacity, and irreverence because cancer is changing. What was once simply a death sentence is slowly becoming, for many, a life sentence." Then we declared: "The art of survivorship is all about how you choose to get busy living."

Under it all was a thick layer of anger. We were done feeling invisible, done being treated like a footnote. To our AYA friends, we declared:

"Welcome to the community you didn't know you needed, where it doesn't matter if you or someone you care about is bald, infertile, metastatic, radioactive, missing a boob, a nut, a vital organ, or just cray from chemo brain. There are no judgments here. Just friends and peers who 'get it' because they already 'got it'."[13]

It was the movement for the times. But times would eventually change.

5 We the Advocates

My dad has always said that the secret to life could be unlocked through three steps:

1. Clean up nice.
2. Make it look good. (In other words, fake it 'til you make it.)
3. Never look under the hood.

These are the nuts and bolts that kept Stupid Cancer going from the moment I launched it. There was so much work to do, and I winged it much of the time, especially in the beginning. I was moving fast and breaking things before that was even the hot new slogan. I was a living, walking "Think Different" Apple commercial about "the crazy ones, the misfits, the rebels, the troublemakers."

When I first entered the advocacy universe, the term "adolescent and young adult cancer" (AYA) hadn't even been coined yet to represent those of us under forty who'd had cancer. There were no young adult-specific standards of care, no dedicated medical research, no peer-reviewed, published journal articles. No white papers. No poster sessions. No guidelines. No best practices, fertility rights, medical education, or specialized AYA cancer programs at hospitals. No survivorship initiatives, and few if any, age-appropriate psychosocial support resources. We were creating something from scratch.

For the first four years, Stupid Cancer scraped by. Every dollar that came in went right back into growing the organization, and I didn't even pay myself. Granted, we had minimal expenses, but we could have moved my radio show out of that airless elevator shaft sooner with a little more cash. I leaned on help wherever I could get it. A few creative agencies worked pro bono to build the Stupid Cancer brand through months-long planning exercises. Kenny worked part-time until we were flush with enough money for him to go full-time.

When the money was good, we rebranded, ran that epic conference in Vegas, and, springboarding off legacy media attention, we got down to the business of de-victimizing cancer for young adults. We never set out to cure the disease, never mind that cancer isn't a single disease. We were instead a mental health quality of life movement for young people. I mean, I bet you've never seen the American Cancer Society organize a bar crawl.

We were watchdogs, calling out how much money was being lavished on "old people's cancer," vacuous ads that all looked the same, inflated management salaries, and real estate. We were doing our own thing, and we were doing it in 1,650 square feet in lower Manhattan.

Did we want research and prevention? Sure. But how do you prevent leukemia when you're twenty-two? There's no screening test, no equivalent of "Check your Balls" or "Save the Ta-tas" for many of the kinds of cancers that young adults get. We reality-checked the usual cancer awareness and fundraising bullshit and said simply that we'd like to die less and die better. Really though, we'd like to live longer and much, much better after cancer.

We began with the stark truth: AYA cancer patients had poorer outcomes than other age groups. That's in part because young patients tend to be diagnosed late and undertreated. Young adults have some of the highest uninsured rates (we're invincible!), thereby delaying diagnosis and care, and they're more likely to ignore or minimize symptoms, figuring they'll just "walk it off." Often, their symptoms aren't taken seriously by doctors who might, oh, prescribe Robitussin for a brain tumor, for example, dropping them squarely into what LIVESTRONG's Young Adult Alliance called a "'no man's land' between pediatric and adult oncology."[1]

As much as I throw around the Robitussin line, I don't blame any doctor for missing my diagnosis, because, when it comes to AYA cancer, there's often no way to connect A to B. How do you tie a 21-year-old pianist who can't arpeggiate to a tumor topping off his cerebellum? To begin with, the odds that any college kid has cancer at all is pretty rare. In fact, the incidence of my particular brain tumor, a medulloblastoma, in adults ages nineteen or older is an estimated one patient *per million*.[2] Meanwhile, about one in ten musicians suffer from the symptoms of carpal tunnel syndrome,[3] one of the many diagnoses tossed into my mix before doctors settled on cancer.

I pissed off quite a few folks in the pediatric oncology space with my 2015 *U.S. News & World Report* article, "The End of Pediatric Cancer Research as We Know It."[4] In it, I argued that childhood cancers were hogging research dollars that chased "cure" while ignoring survivors' long-term quality of life:

> "The benefits of pediatric cancer research still end when you're cured. Why? Because pediatric cancer research has not evolved. It's stuck in the world of biology, lab coats, beakers, electron microscopes, chemistry, and tissue samples. It is hung up on 'cure' and not 'life.'"[5]

As if that wasn't enough mouthing off, I also threw in "and please, no more bald kid commercial appeals." That didn't go over well, especially with parents of pediatric cancer patients. Understandably. Yet, I was technically a pediatric cancer survivor asking the behemoth cancer fundraising organizations to start funding the young adult cancer movement for those of us who had survived cancer as kids and suffered the unique long-term physical and psychosocial issues, like financial toxicity and infertility.

In reality, I was carrying the torch for the cancer mavericks who came before me and further clearing the jungle for those who followed. Without them, we'd never have made it to the point where we are today. We'd never have the rights and the sway we have today if they hadn't paved the way for us all.

Cancer Mavericks

Once upon a time, the term "cancer survivors" referred to the people left behind after someone they loved died of cancer.[6] That's because, more often than not, cancer killed. This was before chemotherapy and radiation, back when surgery was the main treatment and immunotherapy was science fiction. Doctors sometimes didn't even tell patients they had cancer, and some people thought it was contagious. Many used a euphemism for "cancer," even calling it "The Big C."

As the numbers of survivors grew, so did advocacy. It changed the experience and the outcomes for many cancer survivors, bringing in support and humanity where it had been absent.

A few years ago, I set out to discover the origins and the history of cancer advocacy and patient rights through an eight-part podcast series called, "The Cancer Mavericks." It identified the rebels who changed the face of survivorship, decade by decade. Here are their stories.

1960s–1970s

As more people began surviving the disease and the US government started funding the War on Cancer, early heroes arose to advocate for the new survivors—the people who made it through the other side of treatments.

The Philanthropist

In 1969, Mary Lasker, philanthropist, health activist, and the third wife of a New York advertising pioneer who'd died of cancer, took out a full-page ad in the *Washington Post* with the headline: "Mr. Nixon: You can cure cancer."[7] The ad claimed that the war against cancer had the support of 100 percent of Americans: "a war in which we lost 21 times more lives last year than we lost in Vietnam last year." She implored the president to fund research for the cure for cancer by America's 200th birthday. "What a holiday that would be!" It included a form that readers could fill out and mail to the president asking for more cancer research funding.

Lasker had spent $26,000 on the ad, which also appeared in the *New York Times* and the *New York Post*. That's more than $200,000 in today's money. The outcome, however, was priceless, as nearly 8,000 letters soon arrived at the White House.[8]

Then, several senators introduced a bill that would become the National Cancer Act, only it was stuck in committee. So Lasker called Ann Landers, the advice columnist who had some 90 million readers across the country—a super influencer of her day—for help. Landers urged her readers to get involved, "to be part of the mightiest offensive against a single disease in the history of our country," by writing to their senators and asking them to pass the National Cancer Act of 1971. Tens of thousands of letters reached senators' offices calling for Congress to pass the bill.[9]

It did, 79 to 1. (Imagine being the sole senator to say, "Nah. Let's not fight cancer.")

But the House of Representatives was another story. Lasker didn't have as much influence there, and independent scientists testified about their skepticism of her promise to cure cancer by America's big b-day in 1976. Still, it passed the House and soon, President Nixon signed it into law, changing the landscape for cancer research by increasing the National Cancer Institute's budget from $182 million to $1 billion in less than a decade.

The War on Cancer had officially begun and survivorship became a goal. Lasker made sure of that. She had told CBS News anchor Edward R. Murrow, "You won't believe this, but less is spent on cancer research than we spend on chewing gum."[10] Then she set out to change that through an awareness campaign that capitalized on one tactic: embarrassing elected officials into compliance. But she didn't—she couldn't—do it alone.

Early on, she approached Sydney Farber, who was working in a musty laboratory in a children's hospital trying to find the cure for childhood leukemia. When he published the results of one of his successful studies in *The New England Journal of Medicine*, Lasker approached him to serve as the medical expert behind her messaging.

The prevailing wisdom among doctors in the 1950s and 60s was that you could cure cancer only with surgery. Medicine wouldn't work. But Farber had proven that some blood cancers responded to chemotherapy, and together with Lasker, they'd show Congress how cancer funding could improve survival rates overall.

It's *how* they went about getting this message and the support of voters that was so completely new: through advertising that encouraged people to flood Congress with letters. She was the widow of an advertising mogul, after all. Then she added some public relations, through Ann Landers' popular column, and the bill became unstoppable, putting the power of tax dollars behind cancer research for the first time.

The Reporter and the Surgeon

In 1974, Rose Kushner, a mom of three and a reporter for the *Baltimore Sun*, found a lump in her breast during a Saturday night bath. This was the same year that First Lady Betty Ford and Second Lady "Happy" Rockefeller both announced they had breast cancer. The treatment for both women was radical mastectomy.

So Kushner did what any good reporter would do with a new, scary diagnosis: She researched mastectomy and found not much of anything. She went through the stacks at the National Institutes of Health (NIH), made calls, and asked questions. She discovered that the protocol at the time was for the breast surgeon to decide mid-procedure whether or not to perform a mastectomy. That meant that patients went to sleep not knowing whether they'd be missing a breast or both when they woke up. Some women would even end up with radical mastectomies, where the breast, surrounding lymph nodes, plus chest wall muscles, would be removed.

This had been the prevailing treatment, the standard of care, for all types of breast cancer since the 1890s when a surgeon named William Halsted began advocating for the procedure. What Kushner discovered is that nobody had questioned his solution for eighty years. There were no control groups, just Halsted's patients, who all got mastectomies.

Kushner was pissed off, and rightfully so. She searched for a surgeon who'd break ranks and consider a different approach. She called nineteen surgeons and was yelled at or hung up on or both. Some told her that patients shouldn't tell them how to be doctors. Others said she was playing Russian Roulette by not removing her breast.

She found a doctor who'd sign a contract not to remove her breast while she was under anesthesia, but, it turns out, he was convinced it wasn't cancer anyhow and figured he wouldn't have to make that call. Except it was cancer, and that surgeon marched up to Kushner's husband mid-surgery and barked, "She has cancer. She's probably going to die," and then stomped out of the room.

Kushner went on to have a modified mastectomy, which left her lymph nodes and chest muscles intact. In her 1975 book, *Breast Cancer: A Personal History and Investigative Report*, she wrote, "So, in most instances, a woman going to sleep for a simple biopsy does not know whether she will wake up with two breasts or one."[11]

She'd go on to co-found the Breast Cancer Advisory Center telephone hotline to help patients understand their diagnoses and treatment options. She reportedly attended medical conferences in her capacity as a journalist and questioned doctors' data in front of the entire room. She also claimed that the American Medical Association was "hiding important information from the public."[12]

This didn't go over well among doctors, an overwhelmingly male group during the "doctor as God" era, as she was both a patient and a woman. And yet, the National Institutes of Health put her on a breast cancer panel, the only speaker without an MD after her name.

A Pittsburgh surgeon named Dr. Bernie Fisher took notice and believed that what Kushner was saying about breast cancer surgery was probably right. He pushed for clinical trials and made an incredible discovery: Lumpectomy, when a localized tumor is removed from the breast, was often as effective as mastectomy. It was the beginning of tremendous change for breast cancer survivors, and it all started because one patient challenged the status quo.

The 1980s

By the eighties, more people were talking about cancer, and more were surviving it. But surviving didn't necessarily mean thriving. In those days, a cancer diagnosis could cost you your job, your health insurance, and your community, because support that survivors needed wasn't always offered. Cancer doctors often behaved as though survivors were lucky to be alive and therefore, they shouldn't ask for anything more.

But a few cancer survivors believed they had rights, and they weren't afraid to fight for them. The country had just been through a cultural upheaval that gave rise to women's health activists who protested an all-male Senate hearing on birth control. The Black Panthers stood up against health disparities in their neighborhoods that had led to more cancer deaths among Black patients than whites. In New York, a group of Puerto Rican activists called the Young Lords were fighting deplorable conditions at Lincoln Hospital in the Bronx.

All of this churned up the perfect storm that would give rise to cancer advocacy in the 1980s.

The Physician-Survivor and the Alumni Organizer

Fitzhugh "Fitz" Mullen was among the doctors who worked with the Young Lords to occupy that hospital in the Bronx. He wrote about his experiences in a memoir called *White Coat, Clenched Fist*, which addressed what he saw as a lack of humanity in medicine.

Then he became a patient. At thirty-two, married with a three-year-old daughter, he was diagnosed with a tumor in his chest, an anaplastic primary seminoma, a type of testicular cancer that had spread. He wrote about his experience in "Seasons of Survival: Reflections of a Physician with Cancer," in a 1985 issue of *The New England Journal of Medicine*, in which he defined three specific stages of survival. In "acute survival," you're fighting for your life and enduring treatments. In "extended survival," you're in remission or watchful waiting, fearful of recurrence and limited by the effects of treatments. In "permanent survival," it's "the phenomenon we usually call 'cure'" when, he writes, the patient "is indeed a survivor," a "Humpty Dumpty idea of 'good as new'."[13]

He said that though cancer survival rates had doubled in twenty-five years, "we have done very little in a concerted and well-planned fashion to investigate and address the problems with survivors." So, when he moved into extended survival, he started to address what he called the "DMZ" or "purgatory" of survivorship, providing a name and a definition for what thousands of survivors like him were experiencing.[14]

Katherine Logan was one of those survivors. After she endured cervical cancer and the radiation and hysterectomy that came with it, she created a new idea: the patient support group. It was a line in Fitz' survival essay that caught her eye: "What is needed is a consumer network—really an alumni association—of cancer survivors, with meetings, newsletters, and periodicals."[15]

Katherine began putting together a cancer alumni association, starting by writing to Fitz about it and then sending letters to dozens of organizations and people who worked with survivors, inviting them to join a national coalition. They convened in Albuquerque for a weekend-long meeting that would become known as the Constitutional Convention of the National Cancer Survivorship movement. Together, they'd change the semantics of cancer. No longer were patients "cancer victims." Working together with physicians including Fitz, oncology nurses, community activists, and disability attorneys, they developed the National Coalition for Cancer Survivorship (NCCS), now Cancer Nation, to reshape how society views cancer survivors.

The 1990s

In the final decade of the century, cancer survivors were more freely sharing information and their own stories. The NCCS realized they had a problem. They had a hard time reaching poor, rural, and minority communities where survivorship resources were particularly scarce. Early cancer detection and timely treatment were often hindered by poverty and a lack of health insurance, reducing survival rates. Summon the Cancer Mavericks.

The Navigator

In the late 1980s, Dr. Harold P. Freeman, who'd lent his hand to try to improve breast cancer survival rates at Harlem Hospital decades earlier, became the president of the American Cancer Society. He used his national platform to address cancer as it relates to poverty and race, creating a patient navigator program that helped marginalized patient populations find their way through the system.

Not only did it help patients, it helped hospitals. For instance, one hospital in the Bronx had experienced a 95 percent no-show rate for colon cancer screenings. With the new navigator program, however, that rate plummeted to 5 percent. By 2000, Harlem Hospital's five-year breast cancer survival rate had jumped from 39 percent to 70 percent.

The program was so successful, it became a national model, with President George W. Bush signing the Patient Navigator Outreach and Chronic Disease Prevention Act of 2005 to provide funding for hiring and training patient navigators.

Freeman told the Cancer History Project to think of patient navigation as a mile relay race. The four runners are navigators, each carrying and passing off the baton, which represents the patient. Each runner takes the "baton" to the next test, surgery, chemotherapy, etc. "It's not over until you carry that patient across the finish line. And that's the idea of patient navigation."[16]

The Visionary

Ellen Stovall was one of my mentors (see Chapter 4) and a force for good. Diagnosed with stage IV Hodgkin's lymphoma the same year that the National Cancer Act was passed, she wasn't eligible for a clinical trial because she had a menstrual cycle, a factor that barred many women from cancer research at the time. She had the traditional course of chemo and radiation and achieved remission until she had a recurrence in the 1980s.

In those days, the survival rate for Hodgkin's wasn't as high as it is today, and Ellen longed to connect with other patients with the same cancer. Yet even in metropolitan Washington DC, where she was treated, there was a lack of survivorship support, and she was dismayed. Then she found a pamphlet for the newly formed NCCS and attended her first assembly in Albuquerque.

By 1991, she'd become the NCCS Chair of the Assembly, and by the next year, she was looking for office space in DC so the organization could have a greater impact on national cancer policy and research funding. Soon, Ellen took over as Executive Director, becoming a compelling advocate for cancer survivors.

Ellen's personal story lent credence to her messaging. She understood how the healthcare system made it difficult for cancer survivors to access care. When her husband started his own business, their family lost the healthcare coverage they had through his former job. But when they tried to buy their own policy, Ellen had to contact ten insurance companies to find one that would cover her because she was a cancer survivor. Remember, this was before the Affordable Care Act made it illegal to reject healthcare applicants or charge higher rates based on pre-existing conditions. Back then, the individual market simply wasn't a friendly place for people who'd had cancer.

Ellen co-wrote an NCCS report on the pressing needs of cancer survivors. It included a Declaration of Principles that called for quality care, quality of life, rights to healthcare insurance, autonomy, psychosocial support, follow-up care, communication, clinical trials, and long-term support.[17]

The report led to the creation of the National Cancer Institute's Office of Survivorship, a monumental step forward because, for the first time, the focus extended beyond "cure" to "care." Her vision for getting the country's attention was through a march on Washington, a star-studded event that would bring together cancer organizations from around the country. According to the Cancer History Project, *the San Francisco Examiner* reported, "Cancer advocacy is nothing new. What's different is the attempt by The March organizers to marshal the country's eight million cancer survivors into one supergroup."[18]

Some 700 organizations and upwards of 200,000 people marched on that day in the fall of 1998, some of them famous, including Vice President Al Gore, model Cindy Crawford, General Norman Schwarzkopf, skater Scott Hamilton, and Queen Noor of Jordan. Ellen took to the podium and declared, "We are the faces of cancer. We are real. And we are not going away."[19] They'd pulled off one of the largest cancer advocacy events in US history, leading to increased funding for NIH cancer research and the National Cancer Institute.

Her work to frame cancer as a civil rights issue helped lead to the American Disabilities Act in 1990, which provided legal protections for cancer survivors and people with other disabilities.

Ellen kept on fighting until her death in 2016 from a heart condition related to her cancer treatment. The march she spearheaded was a watershed moment for cancer advocacy, one that would shape the movement into the twenty-first century.

The 2000s

By 2000, the five-year survival rate for all cancers had reached 64 percent, up from 50 percent a quarter century earlier.[20] But what did survivorship look like? After I achieved remission in 1996, nobody offered physical therapy to me, a concert pianist with troubles arpeggiating. Nobody suggested that I talk to a social worker about the unique challenges I faced as a 22 year-old on COBRA, trying to get my first job out of college. Nobody talked to me about nutrition to help regain my autoimmune function.

No, I'm not bitter . . . .

After cancer treatments end and you ring the bell and celebrate, it's still not over for the patient. And in the 2000s, there was a lot that needed to be done to make life better for the growing number of cancer survivors.

The Badass MD

Dr. Patricia Ganz is a medical oncologist and a badass. Among the founding members of the NCCS, she's spent four decades researching the late effects of cancer and teaching at UCLA. She also served as a board member of the National Cancer Institute Board of Scientific Advisors and the American Society of Clinical Oncology (ASCO), and she received an American Cancer Society Medal of Honor. She believes work starts when cancer treatments end.

"The physical harm we do to people in order to cure the cancer is quite profound," she told "Cancer Mavericks," adding that survivorship is about helping someone adjust to the "new normal."[21]

Several reports promoted an organized approach to monitoring the health of survivors. The National Academy of Sciences report, "From Cancer Patient to Cancer Survivor: Lost in Transition," called for a "Survivorship Care Plan," which included care coordination between primary care doctors and oncologists.[22] Dr. Ganz chaired a report by the National Academy of Medicine that sounded the alarm about the need for better survivorship care. Finally, the medical community was beginning to address cancer patients and survivors as whole people with issues beyond the disease.

She went on to chair UCLA's LIVESTRONG Survivorship Center of Excellence, explaining, "Oncologists often have no idea what happens to patients when they finish treatment."[23] Dr. Ganz pushed for a written survivorship plan and a process to match. She told *Cancer Today*, "In the old days, doctors were just so happy to have somebody survive. They didn't worry about how [treatment] affected people afterward."[24] Thanks to Dr. Ganz, now they do.

The Young Adult Survivors

When Heidi Adams was twenty-six years old, she was diagnosed with Ewing's sarcoma, a rare cancer that grows in and around the bones. She went from traveling and bartending to the oncology wing of the hospital. She tried to write an irreverent newsletter that would capture the dark sense of humor her generation had come to rely on à la *South Park* and *Beavis and Butthead.*

"It came back, like, all syrupy and inoffensive," she told "Cancer Mavericks." "We were like, 'I don't think that's gonna work.'"[25] She went on to create a website for young adult cancer patients called Planet Cancer, acknowledging the new world every young cancer patient enters. It featured irreverent top ten lists such as "10 Signs

You've Joined a Cheap HMO. Number One: the only expense covered 100 percent is embalming." They sold merch, including T-shirts that said "Planet Cancer: We've done drugs Keith Richards never even heard of."

"Humor makes things less terrifying," Heidi told us. "If you can laugh at something, it loses power over you."[26] Planet Cancer's website featured message boards and offered retreats for young people with cancer, because in the hospital, it's rare to find another young patient like you.

One of those patients was Doug Ulman, an NCAA Division 1 college soccer player. The summer before his sophomore year at Brown University in 1996, he discovered a tumor in the cartilage of his ribs, a chondrosarcoma. Within a year, he'd also be diagnosed with malignant melanoma—twice. When he returned to school, he struggled to find support and answers to the problems that young adult cancer survivors face, including returning to studies, dating, and sports. He founded the Ulman Cancer Fund for Young Adults and distributed 20,000 copies of the foundation's guidebook, *NO WAY, It Can't Be.*

By the 2000s, the foundation had raised more than $3 million, launching patient navigation programs, publishing survivors' stories in *My Way*, and opening new offices. In time, the Ulman Cancer Fund awarded scholarships to young adults, and the Ulman House provided free housing for young adult cancer patients and their caregivers near major hospitals in East Baltimore.

Meanwhile, perhaps the most famous young adult cancer survivor of the times, Lance Armstrong, got a seat at the table of the president's cancer panel. Armstrong, a testicular cancer survivor, had risen to fame with multiple Tour de France titles, and he'd founded what would become LIVESTRONG. Then Nike stepped in and designed the now-famous yellow wristbands, funding the first five million.[27] The hottest accessory ultimately raised millions of dollars. But there was a problem: young adult cancer survival rates hadn't budged in a quarter century.

The Lance Armstrong Foundation worked with the NCI to publish a report called "Closing the Gap," calling for research and care specific to adolescents and young adults with cancer. The foundation formed the Young Adult Alliance, which brought together researchers, doctors, and advocates, including Heidi and Doug. Over the next few years, they raised more than a hundred million dollars for survivorship[28] and acquired Heidi's Planet Cancer.

But then Lance, who'd won seven Tour de France titles in a row, admitted to allegations of doping. He was asked to step down, and Nike pulled its sponsorship of LIVESTRONG. Worst of all, support for cancer survivorship took a hit when Lance's reputation did.

This was the decade that began with NBC's Katie Couric undergoing a colonoscopy live on the *Today* show. For Katie, the issue was immensely personal as her husband, Jay Monahan, had died of colon cancer just two years earlier, at age forty-two. We watched as she drank the gallon of prep—"Bottoms up . . . so to speak"—and press her doctor for plenty of sedation, which she must have gotten because she asked mid-test, "You didn't put the scope in yet?"[29]

After her segment aired, there was a 20 percent increase in colonoscopies nationwide—the Katie Couric effect. Eight years later, she'd co-found Stand Up to Cancer with my friend Laura Ziskin (see Chapter 4), using celebrity to draw attention and hundreds of millions of dollars that helped fund research for nine new cancer therapies that were approved by the FDA, for blood, breast, colorectal, ovarian, and pancreatic cancers.[30]

The Native American Advocate

When Mary P. Lovato, a member of the Santo Domingo Pueblo, a federally recognized Native American tribe in northern New Mexico, was diagnosed with acute leukemia in 1987, she didn't tell her family. In those days, in that region, a cancer diagnosis was something you kept to yourself. But her doctor encouraged her to bring her family to the hospital so he could explain her condition to them.

They wanted to support her, so they tested their bone marrow, and her older sister matched for a transplant.

Lovato soon traveled 800 miles to UCLA for treatment. That's when she met Dr. Linda Burhansstipanov, the founder and president of the American Indian Cancer Research Corporation, which fights to lower the incidence of cancer and improve survival rates among indigenous people.

Most healthcare for the indigenous comes from the Indian Health Service (IHS), a federal agency that provides healthcare to American Indians and Alaska Natives. But when Lovato was diagnosed with cancer, there were no IHS oncology centers near her home in New Mexico, so she had to get her treatment in another state. When she got home, people in her community were scared that her illness was contagious. It was as though if she even said the word "cancer," she'd spread it through the community.

So, Lovato started a support group in the Pueblo. At first, no one showed up, but she didn't give up. For three years, she and other volunteers ran support groups for cancer survivors, without pay or financial assistance, believing they could save lives. Eventually, Dr. Stepanov helped them secure funding from the IHS. This was a huge deal, because the IHS has been seriously underfunded by Congress, with about $4,000 allocated per patient compared to Medicare's $13,000 each.[31]

When Lovato started her advocacy work, cancer was low on the list of prioritized health conditions that the IHS could cover. Chemotherapy and radiation for just one patient could wipe out a tribe's entire IHS budget. Yet the incidence of leukemia and bone cancer is higher in Native areas near abandoned uranium mines, where elevated radiation levels have created cancer clusters.

Lovato's advocacy included training Native Americans to become navigators who accompany patients to appointments, which improved the relationships between doctors and the community. She also helped to destigmatize cancer among the indigenous, showing that it isn't contagious or a curse.

For twenty-three years, Lovato survived leukemia, bone cancer, and kidney cancer before she passed away in 2008. She is remembered for her visionary efforts to improve treatment and support for the Native people.

The Disparities Breaker

In 2006, Maimah Karmo knew something wasn't right with her body. Growing up in Liberia, she was familiar with physical health because her mother was the head of the country's nursing association. Her mother was the one who taught her how to do the breast self-exam that would end up saving her life.

At thirty-two, Maimah was living in the Washington, DC area with her own young daughter when she discovered a lump in her breast while showering. A mammogram revealed two lumps, so she was referred to a breast surgeon who told her she had no evidence of cancer. "Come back when you're older," she said. "Don't worry about it." Her own doctor thought she was "too young" for cancer, just one reason why AYA cancers are so often diagnosed late.

But Maimah couldn't shake the feeling that something was wrong. She pushed for a biopsy, which would lead to the truth: She had stage II triple negative breast cancer. If she hadn't made that discovery when she did, her result would have been life-threatening. She told "Cancer Mavericks" that her mother's patient advocacy empowered her to do the same for her own health. "If I hadn't seen my mom talk to doctors eyeball to eyeball my whole life, I would be dead today."[32]

When she began treatment, she swore she'd do whatever she could to help others with breast cancer. She'd go on to found the Tigerlily Foundation to support and empower young women with breast cancer.

She's also committed to reducing disparities in breast cancer survival rates. That's because Black had a 40 percent higher death rate than white patients twenty years ago. They aren't as likely to be offered genetic testing or clinical trials; the enrollment for Black women was just 3 percent.

Maimah told "Cancer Mavericks" that clinical trials work on a reimbursement basis, so that patients pay up front for transportation costs. "If you're missing work, who pays for those lost wages or a lost job?"

Such disparities not only affect clinical trials, but they also create a lack of access to insurance and transportation, which can create a barrier to earlier diagnosis and care. Maimah worked to end systemic barriers and disparities by eliciting a pledge by pharmaceutical companies to design and build clinical trials that take the special concerns of marginalized communities into consideration. Tigerlily Foundation's inclusion pledge has more than 12,000 signatures so far.

Selma Schimmel

Diagnosed with breast cancer at twenty-eight in the early 1980s, Selma found few support systems for young adults with cancer. She founded Vital Options International, a global health foundation that addresses health disparities by supporting patients' financial, educational, and advocacy needs. Selma took no shit from anyone, and she was crucial to my success as an AYA cancer advocate. She'd set up terrestrial radio live interviews at oncology conferences and later offered me my own show. Honestly, if I were a decade older and I wasn't already dating my future wife, Jessica, I'd have asked Selma to marry me. She fought for patient-centered research and a voice in clinical care trial design and was a trailblazer in AYA cancer advocacy, all the while fighting cancer multiple times until her death in 2014 at age fifty-nine.

Advocacy Spreads

Cancer survivorship advocacy has come a long way in the past sixty years, and it's thanks in no small part to all the Cancer Mavericks who've challenged the status quo, sticking up for what matters for all cancer survivors and their families.

But what worked so well for so many years requires a shift in philosophies and action to bring patients what they need most now: consumer protections. It's why I made the decision to leave Stupid Cancer and head in a different direction that changes the face of cancer advocacy, and it needs you to succeed.

6 We the Consumers

When you're first diagnosed, you're in the "Oh Shit Window" when you are most likely to get taken advantage of by various corners of the American healthcare system. The trick to surviving sounds simple: *Don't try to fix it. Rig it.* But you've got to figure out how real fast, because this is your Diarrhea Moment. Take care of it right away or else you could wind up getting billed for something you're not obligated to pay for, stuck with a doctor you hate, discover that the treatment you're about to start isn't covered by your insurance, and other assorted bullshit.

The "healthcare consumers" who understand that the system isn't broken but instead, deliberately stacked against them, often fare the best because they know the truth: the American healthcare system was designed to prioritize profits, not patients. Your insurance company isn't set up to have your best interest in mind. If you are not demonstrating profit for their shareholders, if your MRI or stem cell transplant or cutting-edge immunotherapy is siphoning off their quarterly earnings, then you might end up in Healthcare Purgatory, where every denial is revenue. While you're stuck on hold with your insurance company listening to the Doobie Brothers' "What a Fool Believes," understand this: You can rig this system if you know how.

The good news is that there are people, organizations, and information to guide you through it if you aren't afraid to ask for help. Today, there are many resources available, and the internet makes it easy to access them. It helps that people no longer whisper "cancer," as though if they said it out loud they'd catch it. We've stopped being a society that hushes cancer or its survivors. It also helps that there have been decades of cancer advocacy that have not only provided you with rights we didn't have before, but also emotional support resources.

Though I'm about to share with you what I consider the top five of these resources, this is no time to leave it all up to someone else, but you might want to at least trust your doctor. I like to quote my friend Kris Carr of "Crazy Sexy Cancer" who said that when you're first diagnosed, you have to act like the leader of a small business, the "CEO of Save My Ass Technologies, Inc."[1] When she was diagnosed with a rare and incurable sarcoma in 2003, she assembled the best team she could to support her health, and she's still going strong.

That team isn't just you and your oncologist. It can include people who help you navigate your care, understand your diagnosis and evaluate your treatments, fight denials from your insurance company, teach you how to talk about your diagnosis with your kids, explain your rights at work, get financial assistance, locate and apply for a clinical trial, coordinate support, and organize it all.

It's okay to hire and fire people from your team because your care should be on your terms, though that's easier said than done where insurance is involved. And let's shout this one from the hospital rooftop: GoFundMe shouldn't have to be your team's designated hitter. But let's face it, it's where paying for big healthcare bills has landed in this country right now.

Once you have the diagnosis and, hopefully, a second opinion that confirms it, it's time to step onto the board game that is cancer and prepare for the pitfalls and booby traps that you may come upon along the way. I'm focusing on insurance, work/employment, medical debt, and clinical trials, though that's by no means an exhaustive list.

Keep in mind that American healthcare is going through a tremendous shift, and I hesitate to supply government resources, especially considering the Centers for Disease Control and Prevention (CDC) is getting gutted as I write this. But there are and always have been cancer advocates who step up to support and protect us. I've chosen five that I think are among the best and sprinkled them into this chapter like magical fairy dust for cancer patients.

The Mother of All Healthcare Fuckery

The very first question that you'll be asked when you become a patient is "Do you have insurance?" or, more likely, "What kind of insurance do you have?" Because if you don't have insurance, you automatically have far fewer options in this country.

Your health insurance plan is sort of like boarding groups for airlines. The more comprehensive your coverage, the more likely you're sitting in First or Business Class with a nice blanket and extra snacks. Meanwhile, the people with high-deductible HMOs from the bronze-level Affordable Care Act (ACA) plans are sitting in the last rows, forced to check their bags at the gate, while they endure getting elbowed in the head by people in line to the bathrooms.

You may get your insurance through your employer, a union, the ACA, the government, or an association plan. (I'm leaving several government-sponsored plans off this list, which I explain below.) Here's my unscientific ranking of America's insurance options, from "least worst" to *ugh*. The higher the ranking, the less douchebaggery you're likely to deal with during treatments and beyond:

1. **PPO—Preferred Provider Organization.** The PPO is often the plan used to attract big talent to big companies. If you're in finance, a tech bro, a healthcare worker, a member of a big-time labor union, or a tenured university professor, (or you're married to any of these), you probably have a PPO, and it's likely heavily subsidized by your employer. Lucky you. You can

see a specialist without a referral, among other perks. On the ACA, there are typically a handful of PPOs, and they tend to be pricey because they provide flexibility to see out-of-network providers.

2. **Medicare.** If you're 65 or older, this is the sweet government plan you've been paying into your entire career and now it's yours. As of 2026, there's a deductible of $1,736 and coinsurance for hospital stays (Part A), but this is the closest thing America has to universal healthcare, at least for our seniors, and most doctors and hospitals accept it. Traditional Medicare rarely requires prior authorizations though they're seeping in through Medicare Advantage, an optional plan offered by private healthcare companies (see Chapter 8). I hope Medicare is still there when I get to 65. There are all sorts of add-on plans, or "Parts," and the rules seem to change frequently. I'm no expert, but there are plenty of them on TikTok if you're looking for guidance.

3. **EPO—Exclusive Provider Organization.** In an EPO, referrals from your primary care physician (PCP) for specialists are not required, and you can see anyone in-network you'd like, but the plan doesn't cover out-of-network providers. So, unless they're subject to the No Surprises Act, like an assistant surgeon or emergency department doctor (see Chapter 7), you're stuck with the bill. EPOs are cheaper than PPOs for employers but they tend to provide more choice for employees than HMOs (see below).

4. **POS—Point of Service.** Part PPO, part HMO, a POS means you have to get referrals from your PCP to see specialists. Still, you might be able to get a blanket referral to your oncologist, so you don't have to visit your primary first every damn time you go for cancer care. If you want to go to an out-of-network doctor though, you might have paperwork and phone calls in your future.

5. **HDHP—High-Deductible Health Plan.** These are low-premium, high-deductible plans popular with younger and healthier people who don't use their health insurance that much. They often come with Health Savings Accounts (HSA) that let you put aside pre-tax money for medical costs, like eyeglasses and medication co-pays. But if you get sick, this plan might not be the best choice. For instance, you could be on the hook for upwards of $3,300 for deductibles for a family, depending on the annual rule set by the IRS, plus an out-of-pocket maximum of $16,600.

6. **HMO—Health Maintenance Organization.** A good half of ACA plans are HMOs, and smaller employers like them because they're cheaper than PPOs. With most HMOs, you can only use in-network providers except for emergencies, and your PCP becomes the gatekeeper of all your care, though some plans don't require referrals,[2] so read the fine print.

7. **AHP—Association Health Plans.** This is when a group of employers or trade groups band together through an association, pooling resources to buy coverage as though they're a large employer. These existed before the ACA, sometimes providing coverage for individuals like freelance writers. The Trump administration expanded rules through the Department of Labor in 2018 that made it easier for individuals to join an AHP, creating competition with the ACA. For instance, AHPs can allow you to cross state lines for care, which some states, such as New Jersey, stopped offering on the ACA. But, depending on your state, some plans can exclude benefits, like maternity care, that the ACA requires. That's because they are designed to exclude or limit costly care, like certain cancer drugs, depending on state law. So if you're in a more permissive state, such as Florida, rather than a more regulated one, like New York, an AHP might be able to bypass consumer protections, thereby excluding you from some benefits. Read the fine print.

Government Assistance Plans

There are several government plans designed to help low-income citizens, the US military, and marginalized groups.

- **Medicaid:** I'm not ranking Medicaid on my bulleted list because it's a safety net for low-income Americans who can't afford private health insurance. And it's been "DOGEd," slashed with historic funding cuts of nearly $1 trillion over a decade, a victim of the One Big Beautiful Bill. It's the biggest source of health funding for the disabled and elderly,[3] and, along with the Children's Health Insurance Program (CHIP), it's the largest single insurer of children, covering nearly half of all US children.[4]
- **Veterans Affairs Health Care (VA):** The VA is not really insurance, but a government-funded healthcare system that's run by the US Department of Veterans Affairs. Eligible veterans don't pay monthly premiums, but there can be copays depending on your income level, disability, and military service history.
- **TRICARE:** This health insurance program, run by the Department of Defense, functions like private insurance for active-duty military service members, retirees, National Guard and Reserve members, and their families.
- **Indian Health Services (IHS):** The IHS provides healthcare for American Indians and Alaska Natives who are members of federally recognized tribes.

Your Employer-Sponsored Health Plan

If you get your insurance through your employer, you need to know if it's self-funded or fully insured because they are regulated differently:

- **Self-funded:** The employer takes the risk and Employee Retirement Income Security Act (ERISA) rules apply to protect employees from plan mismanagement. You might have to fight your own employer and, as the late Marshall Allen wrote in "Never Pay the First Bill," "Your employer is not necessarily your friend."[5] About two-thirds of employees are covered by self-funded plans.[6]

- **Fully insured**: The insurer takes the risk and state rules apply.

Pick a Card: Prior Auth or Denial

Assuming you have some sort of insurance coverage, the game of Healthcare Fuckery comes with two key ways to impede your ability to interfere with your insurance company's profits: Prior authorization (see Chapter 2) or claim denial. Think of them like Monopoly's Chance and Community Chest, where the cards can keep you from advancing in the game and you do not pass Go or collect $200, so to speak.

Let's say your doctor wants you to get a PET scan to determine if your cancer is still in remission, but your insurance company stamps it with a giant red NO, or whatever the e-version is. Robot or human, it doesn't matter who didn't grant it. You're not getting that scan unless you pay for it yourself, and it can cost thousands of dollars.

Insurance companies fail to grant prior auths for a variety of reasons, including: "medical necessity," paperwork mistakes, and plan guidelines, which may require you to try and fail other procedures or medicines first.

According to the AMA, 80 percent of prior auth appeals[i] succeed, so why not fight it?[7] Most people don't, with just about 0.2 percent appealing their denials.[8] The process is slightly different with each healthcare company, so read up on their requirements, but chances are you'll need a copy of your Explanation of Benefits (EOB), which provides the reason for the denial, your diagnosis, and your CPT

---

[i]These stats are specifically about Medicare Advantage plans.

codes, the AMA's coding system for diagnoses and procedures. There are a few ways to appeal:

- **Peer-to-peer review.** If your prior authorization was denied as medically unnecessary, your doctor may request a peer-to-peer review with a doctor who works for your insurance company. Don't expect that doctor to practice the same kind of medicine as yours or to have any experience with whatever medical test or procedure that's being denied. Yes, that means you could wind up with a urologist reviewing whether your brain cancer really needs that newly approved, one-of-a-kind therapy that targets mutated genes to slow tumor growth, but hey, at least you have insurance?
- **Appeal letter.** To file an appeal, you'll need to ask your doctor to write and submit a letter on your behalf within sixty days of your denial. They'll know what needs to accompany the letter, but usually it's your consult notes and test results. Adding copies of peer-reviewed studies that support your appeal can also be helpful.[9] Some larger doctors' offices have dedicated staff, such as nurse navigators or insurance coordinators, to fight denials, while others leave it up to the doctor to carve out time each day. If it's urgent, your doctor can request an expedited appeal if they include valid reasons for the rush.
- **Personal narrative.** Appeals, so far, are read by humans. Tug at their heart strings with your own letter explaining why you need the test, procedure, treatment, or medication, including your illness' effect on your quality of life. Be respectful; you might want to write the angry version first just to get it out of your system and then edit accordingly.

It's likely that these must be submitted by fax. Remember fax machines? Your insurer is required to provide a decision for a prior auth denial within 30 days. Expedited appeals must be decided within four business days and can be delivered verbally, but a written notice must be provided within 48 hours.[10]

If your prior auth is denied again, you can appeal a second time or, in some cases, request an external review, when a third party determines any adverse effects based on "medical necessity, appropriateness, healthcare setting, level of care, or effectiveness of a covered benefit."[11] Sometimes, an external review is used for denials related to an experimental or investigational treatment. Each state has its own rules for whether you qualify and how long the review should take, so check yours.

We the Support

#1: Patient Advocate Foundation
When Nancy Davenport-Ennis lost a friend to breast cancer who was also battling her own insurance company, she launched this nonprofit organization to provide case management services, free one-on-one support for resolving insurance denials, accessing disability benefits, and addressing financial hardship. They offer comprehensive guides to navigating prior auths, among other helpful information. (patientadvocate.org).

After-the-Fact Claim Denials

The reasons for claim denials can include: failing to secure a prior auth, out-of-network physician, incorrect billing codes, missed claim deadlines, inaccurate patient information, and faulty claim information, among others.[12]

How do you file an appeal on a claim denial? It's similar to a prior auth denial appeal, and it depends on the reason for the denial and your insurance company's protocol. Generally speaking, it goes like this:

- **Appeal letter.** If there were errors in the original claim, such as coding mistakes, a revised claim is submitted with the correct information. If your claim was deemed medically unnecessary, your doctor writes a letter explaining why the procedure or treatment is medically necessary, and includes medical records, lab results, consult notes, etc. You may also write your own letter, and it should include your member ID, the EOB reference number, and your date of birth. Explain your diagnosis, the symptoms, your physician's name, and the reason your doctor says you needed the treatment or procedure. Attach any documentation, such as medical records and journal articles. There's a time limit for appeals, typically about 60 days post-procedure or treatment.

- **External review.** If your appeal for a denial based on medical necessity fails, you might be eligible to order an external review. Each state has its own process, so check yours. Some states don't have a process, so you might need to contact the Department of Health and Human Services (HHS) instead. You'll need a request form, your final denial letter, EOBs, medical records, and a doctor's letter that explains your medical necessity. You have four months after your final denial notice to request an external review.

Make the Robots Work for You

If robots can issue denials, can they help you appeal them? Yes, they can. There's an emerging cottage industry of companies that will help you draft AI–assisted appeal letters. For a fee, they pull relevant details from the insurance plan policies, EOBs, and other documents to wordsmith your appeal for you. Caveat emptor. You can also direct ChatGPT or another AI program to do the work for you, and fast. One blog called AI appeals "technological jujitsu, using the opponent's strength against them," declaring the best news of all: "The robots are finally on our side."[13]

We the Support

#2: Cancer Care

Does it feel like you need a medical degree to understand how to manage cancer treatments? Cancer Care has been taking notes for you. Founded in 1944, the nonprofit offers free support services and information to manage the emotional, practical, and financial challenges of a cancer diagnosis. You can get counseling and guidance from oncology social workers, join a support group, take a workshop, read booklets and fact sheets, and get help with financial assistance.

(cancercare.org).

Who's Paying for All This?

Medical debt continues to be an insidious problem for so many Americans. As of 2021, more than half of all third-party debt collection "tradelines," lingo for credit report accounts, were for medical debt.[14] With an estimated 15 million people expected to lose insurance[15] coverage thanks to the OBBB, some estimates anticipated a 15 percent increase in medical debt, totaling upwards of $50 billion.[16]

No one plans to become a "healthcare consumer." It just happens when you wind up with a diagnosis that costs a lot to treat, and cancer often does. It is fourth in overall annual costs for Americans, at about $200 billion, after Alzheimer's, diabetes, and heart disease and stroke.[17] *The Wall Street Journal* reported that cancer creates financial toxicity with treatments like chemo leading to a "two-fold blow" that can keep people out of work for weeks or months, "with patients losing income and their employer-sponsored health insurance" at the same time.[18]

Here are some ways to protect yourself:

- **Ask for the price up front.** The newish hospital transparency laws (see Chapter 7) allow patients to find out how much tests and procedures will cost. You can use the Fair Health Consumer (fairhealthconsumer.org) cost estimator. Just be sure to get the right CPT codes up front to plug them in.
- **Request itemized bills.** That way you can catch errors, like duplicate charges or being charged for a treatment you never got. Call the billing department to fix or remove errors.
- **Negotiate.** Call patient financial services to ask for discounts. Some of the language you can use includes "prompt-pay discounts," "self-pay/uninsured rate," "charity care," and "financial assistance." Keep in mind that nonprofit hospitals are required by law to offer charity care and financial assistance, and yet, they often don't.
- **Find payment options.** You can finance monthly payments at as low as 0 percent, get a discount for paying a lump sum up front, and arrange hardship discounts if your income qualifies.

We the Support

#3: Dollar For

Many people don't know that most hospitals are required to offer discounts or debt forgiveness for some patients. National nonprofit Dollar For has eliminated more than $100 million in medical debt for patients nationwide. That's especially remarkable considering their own study revealed that more than half of patients reported receiving no information from their hospital about financial assistance. What's more, Black patients were less likely than other races to be approved for charity care.

(dollarfor.org)

Working While Sick

The thing about tying healthcare to work is that when you're sick, it's hard to work. But there are laws and programs designed to help you navigate working (or not working) when you're battling illness, depending on where you're employed. Even when the treatments are over, or at least in maintenance mode, working isn't likely to be exactly as it was before your diagnosis, at least not for a while. You'll probably have doctor's appointments, scans, blood tests, and other medical mayhem affecting your workdays. This is where laws that protect patients will come into play, so brush up on your legal rights as a patient.

If you're self-employed, the rules are different for you. You'll need to determine if you're going to share your diagnosis with clients and customers or keep it to yourself. You may want to delegate work to your employees or, if you're a solopreneur like 80 percent of small businesses,[19] outsource it to trusted colleagues. Consider creating a contract that protects your work from being permanently removed from you.

Current ACA laws prevent health plans from discriminating against you or dropping you for a cancer diagnosis. That said, you'll need to keep up your premium payments through your illness. If your income drops, you may be eligible for Medicaid or disability benefits. And there's always a GoFundMe to help cover medical costs. May the best tribute win. I'm kidding. Maybe, maybe not.

We the Support

#4: Cancer and Careers

Each year, this organization assists about a half million people by providing resources related to cancer and the workplace, helping patients return to work after a diagnosis and treatment. They offer webinars about job searching, balancing work and cancer, and shifting careers, among others, and they lay out how to return to work after treatments. (cancerandcareers.org)

Are Clinical Trials for You?

There are multiple reasons to consider joining a clinical trial, which is a research study to test new treatments, combinations of medications, surgical procedures, radiation techniques, and more. Typically, people join clinical trials when standard therapies stop working, or if they have a rare cancer with few treatment options. For adult cancers, participation is not common, with only about 8 percent of patients participating.[20]

Clinical trials provide access to cutting-edge treatments and promising therapies that might not be widely available for years. For some patients, they're a Hail Mary, a last-ditch effort when the standard therapies fail. National Cancer Institute (NCI)-designated medical centers have the highest participation rate, at about 22 percent.[21] These are teaching and research hospitals in major cities, for the most part.

Understand that routine care costs, like doctor's visits, scans, and bloodwork, will likely be billed to your insurance, so it's important to have good coverage if you sign up for a clinical trial. Out-of-pocket costs like travel are often not covered. Of course, that's part of the reason that there are diversity gaps in trials, with about 83 percent of participants being white.[22]

Your trial might require a prior authorization through your insurance company, so make sure you look into it before you sign on. Some clinical trials have staff who work directly with health plans to get you hooked up. Some federal health insurance will help pay for clinical trial costs, including Medicaid, Medicare, TRICARE, and the Department of Veterans Affairs.[23]

To find a clinical trial, visit ClinicalTrials.gov.

We the Support

#5: Triage Cancer®
This national nonprofit provides free information about the legal and practical issues that cancer patients and their

caregivers face after a diagnosis. They address health insurance coverage, employment and work rights, survivorship care planning, and finances, among others.

"People say to me, 'What's legal about cancer?'" cofounder Monica Bryant told me. "The answer back is almost everything is legal about cancer." This includes the medications a patient has access to, the health insurance they pay for, the rights they have at work, how doctors treat them, estate planning, and finances. "It's all rooted in the law." (triagecancer.org)

Happy Customers

When you begin to shift your perspective from cancer patient at the mercy of the system to consumer who deserves protections just like any other, you begin to see American's healthcare shitshow in an entirely different light. And it will probably piss you off. Once you figure out how to rig it to your personal favor, zoom out for the bigger picture. There's work to do.

7

We the Relentless

In 2019, Jon Stewart ripped Congress a new one because of health-care, or the lack of it. The *Daily Show* host and comedian appeared before a House Judiciary subcommittee on behalf of first responders to deliver what *GQ* called "angry blistering testimony" for "a fight he's clearly grown sick of" about the September 11th Victim Compensation Fund.[1] Behind him were first responders, some of them sick and dying from exposure to toxins at Ground Zero, and they were pissed.

Though Congress had passed the James Zadroga 9/11 Health and Compensation Act in 2010 and renewed it in 2015 for another five years, it hadn't yet been extended. The Never Forget the Heroes Act[2] would have made funding permanent, but Senate Majority Leader Mitch McConnell wouldn't bring it to a vote, and now, the five-year extension was running out.

Stewart didn't hold back when he railed into the committee, explaining that the first responders were there to fight for what's right, asking for funding and yet being treated "like children trick-or-treating, rather than the heroes that they are."[3]

They had seen this before. In the 2000s, they were gaslighted, told that their illnesses had nothing to do with "the pile" of toxic rubble at Ground Zero. Years later, when science proved it was, they were told it's a "New York issue" and anyhow there wasn't enough money. But, as Stewart said, "Al Qaeda didn't shout out 'Death to Tribeca.'"[4] This was about America.

CBS News reported that Stewart had been "disgusted" by the hearing's small turnout by Congressional committee members, calling it an embarrassment and a stain. "You should be ashamed of yourselves for not being here."[5]

"There isn't an empty chair on that stage that didn't tweet out 'Never forget the heroes of 9/11,'" he said. "Setting aside that no American in this country should face financial ruin because of a health issue, certainly 9/11 first responders shouldn't have to decide whether to live or have a place to live."[6]

By all accounts, Stewart and the first responders had all the ingredients to push legislation through Congress much faster than it took: sympathetic heroes who were considered patriots that had stepped up on behalf of their city and their country, represented by a persuasive and famous spokesperson who brought a briefcase full of shame to Congress.

But it took nearly eighteen years after the attacks before the permanent funding was finally signed into law by President Trump, supplying money for 9/11 first responder health benefits through 2090. Was Congress unanimous in their "yea" votes? Nay. Twelve House representatives and two senators, Rand Paul (R-KY) and Mike Lee (R-UT), voted against the bill, with Paul calling for commensurate cuts in other areas to pay for it, all while Senator Kirsten Gillibrand (D-NY) tearfully objected.[7] But they finally had the votes and the president's support. At least, for a while. The World Trade Center Health Program got "DOGEd" in 2025, losing 20 percent of its staff to budget cuts.[8]

Anytime anyone does their part to make healthcare better, most people haven't seen the work that goes behind it when advocates go diving into the bowels of our legislative branch. We get a right we didn't have before or healthcare coverage that's new and we're grateful for the change, but we often have no idea how it got there because it wasn't brought to a public vote. It was all done behind the scenes, and it takes clips from an angry comedian's testimony via C-SPAN to hit social media to get our attention.

But our lives as survivors are much better because of the dogged determination of a few so that we don't have to go "trick-or-treating" for our healthcare. Here are some of the "yeas" that have it for all of us:

Cancer Nation

The second highest grossing movie of 1983 (after *Return of the Jedi*) was about a cancer victim. I'm only using the word "victim" because that's what people called us forty years ago, and it's how *Terms of Endearment* portrayed Debra Winger's character when she was diagnosed with "lumps" under her arm. Could be breast cancer. Could be a blood cancer. The movie never says. You're just supposed to feel sorry for her and then use up all the tissues when she says goodbye to her kids.

Back then, many cancers were a death sentence, and, as I've said, some people even thought cancer was contagious. In fact, the National Coalition for Cancer Survivorship, now Cancer Nation, reported that a woman who finished treatment for laryngeal cancer said that she came back to work to find a film of Lysol blanketing her desk. Others thought that people who'd endured cancer couldn't possibly be as productive as everyone else.[9]

But we weren't and aren't victims. We just got dealt shitty cards. The co-founders knew that. In Chapter 5, I mentioned some of what drove them to meet for the first time, in Albuquerque in the mid-1980s. But it's not until you look closely at their achievements over the decades that you truly begin to understand how their efforts have brought on important and lasting changes that make life better for the cancer survivors formerly known as victims.

Americans with Disabilities Act (ADA)

In 1987, NCCS co-founder and disability rights attorney Barbara Hoffman, JD, testified before a Congressional subcommittee in a "Hearing on Discrimination Against Cancer Victims and the Handicapped." Never mind the dated title. This was the 1980s after all. The purpose of the hearing was to discuss making discrimination against the disabled an unlawful employment practice in all fifty states and in DC.

Hoffman and the NCCS' solution was the Cancer Patients' Employment Rights Act, which would address discrimination against survivors, including insurance companies raising rates or refusing insurance, banks denying loans, and society in general's assumptions that we were all likely to die anyhow so why make any plans at all? Hoffman assured the panel that "there is life after cancer" and it should be filled with equal opportunities under the law. The bill prohibited cancer-based discrimination, and "because discrimination against qualified cancer survivors is a national problem, it requires a federal solution."[10]

The bill was later folded into the ADA, which passed in 1990 and protects individuals with a record of a disability—cancer in remission is considered one—as protected classes. You might bristle at being considered disabled when cancer is in your rearview mirror and you feel like you get by just fine, but remember, back in the 1980s, people used to Lysol our desks, kick us off insurance, and shred our resumés. You have this organization to thank for the fact that no one discriminates against you for surviving cancer.

Cancer Leadership Council

Remember those seventy-odd times that the ACA was attacked (see Chapter 2)? The NCCS joined a coalition of cancer organizations in 2017 to oppose President Trump's American Health Care Act, which sought to repeal and replace the ACA, weakening protections for people with pre-existing conditions. KFF estimated that about six million people with pre-existing conditions would have faced higher healthcare rates under the law,[11] which passed the House of Representatives anyhow. The Congressional Budget Office (CBO) estimated that the law would leave 23 million people uninsured by 2026. And we had no idea a pandemic was around the corner.

The NCCS joined 37 national patient advocacy groups—including Stupid Cancer—to push back, stating that, even though the bill retained some patient protections, "those protections are meaningless to patients if coverage is unaffordable."[12] Ultimately, John McCain (R-AZ) killed the bill with his dramatic thumbs-down vote on the Senate floor (see Chapter 2). The NCCS said of the Trump bill, "This cannot and should not be the way forward in healthcare in America."[13]

DIEP Flap Breast Reconstruction Codes

Sometimes, insurance coverage for cancer and post-cancer treatments comes down to a code on a form. It's the kind of in-the-weeds, insurance billing stuff that only insiders tend to know about. But stick with me, because this one's important if you've ever considered breast reconstruction after mastectomy.

In breast reconstruction surgery, there are several flap procedures. One is called TRAM (Transverse Rectus Abdominis Myocutaneous), and it uses muscle from the abdominal wall and implants to reconstruct the breast.[14] A more advanced, muscle-sparing, microsurgical procedure called DIEP (Deep Inferior Epigastric Perforator), uses a patient's own tissue, which reportedly feels softer and more natural.[15] For a while, these two procedures were coded differently. The less complicated but more invasive TRAM was reimbursed at a lower rate than the more complex and, often, patient-preferred, "gold standard"[16] DIEP. In fact, without insurance, a DIEP flap surgery can cost more than $50,000.[17]

The Centers for Medicare and Medicaid (CMS) were going to let the "S codes" for DIEP flap "sunset" at the end of 2024, so that surgeons would be reimbursed at the lower TRAM rate. The change would affect private insurers as well as Medicare and Medicaid recipients, and *KFF Health News* reported that it was the Blue Cross and Blue Shield Association that first requested the discontinuation of the codes.[18] When CMS decided to do that, "at least two major insurance companies told doctors they would no longer reimburse them under the higher-paying codes," reports *KFF*.[19]

Cancer Nation was among the voices to speak up for maintaining the codes. So, too, did a bipartisan group of lawmakers led by two cancer survivors, Rep. Debbie Wasserman Schultz (D-FL) and Sen. Amy Klobuchar (D-MN), and Cancer Nation CEO Shelley Fuld Nasso who advised CMS at a public meeting that the two surgeries are not equal from a patient perspective.

"As advocates for patients, we weigh in on coverage and reimbursement issues," said Fuld Nasso, "because we know that, in our health care system, what is paid for gets done, and without adequate payment for physicians, patients will not receive the services they need."[20]

In 2024, CMS dropped their plans to eliminate the billing codes. Cancer Nation's vice chair Lisa D. T. Rice told *Stat News*, "We shouldn't have to fight to keep a benefit we've had for nearly two decades, one which is a vital part of quality care."[21] And yet.

Cancer Nation's Fuld Nasso told me that there's no end to cancer advocacy.

"Just because you have a win, it doesn't mean you can stop. You have to keep going. Unfortunately, it's not all linear progress, and we have to keep reminding people why everything we do is so important."

The No Surprises Act

Have you ever been to the ER, only to wind up with an enormous bill for out-of-network care? Maybe you were rushed in by ambulance or perhaps you checked yourself in, finding out later that, though the hospital is in your network, not everyone who treated you is. Maybe you had a follow-up visit with one of the doctors who cared for you in the hospital, yet they're not in-network. Or some out-of-network doctor you never even saw interpreted your CT scan or your lab work. So you were charged for what your insurance wouldn't cover and boy, hospital bills can be a whopper, huh? All of this was a surprise to you, and now you might feel like you could use medical attention.

Well, you're going to love the No Surprises Act, which was signed into law in 2020 and went into effect nationwide in 2022. It protects consumers against "balance billing," when a provider charges the patient the difference between the insurance payout and the total amount for care. Under the No Surprises Act, you can't be balance-billed for emergency medicine, anesthesia, laboratory, pathology, radiology, assistant surgeons, neonatology, hospitalists, or critical care services.[22]

How does it work? Imagine you've had a heart attack and an out-of-network assistant surgeon scrubs in to save your life. Weeks later, you nearly have another heart attack when you get balance-billed for that surgeon. Now, you don't have to imagine it because chances are, the No Surprises Act protects you from these balance billing shenanigans. So, how did we get this legislative gem?

It started with a 2019 bill co-written by a physician-Senator, Bill Cassidy (R-LA). Cassidy used his Dr. Senator powers for good and introduced the bipartisan bill with Senator Maggie Hassan (D-NH), who was accompanied at the State of the Union Address by a constituent who'd been balance-billed $1,600 for a five-minute ER visit from an out-of-network doctor.[23]

It all looks like a bipartisan kumbaya now, but, as with anything healthcare related, Congress wasn't quick to get behind the bill because lobbyists were working hard against it, creating a years-long deadlock. Though 40 percent of Americans were worried about unexpected medical bills in 2018,[24] lobbyists fought the No Surprises Act. Were they lobbyists for doctors and hospitals? Not according to *Kaiser Health News*, who called out private equity and venture capital firms as the voice of opposition.

Lobbyists for Envision Healthcare, a medical staffing company, fought the bill.[25] Who owns Envision, you ask? Kohlberg Kravis Roberts & Co. (KKR), a private equity firm that bought Envision for nearly $10 billion in 2018.[26] See also: TeamHealth, owned by Blackstone. Together, they tried to smother the bill.

To understand why they were so dead set against the act, we need to take to the air–air ambulances. Air ambulance companies are notorious for sending hefty balance bills after they've airlifted your loved one to the hospital. I'm talking $50,000, $60,000 bills.[27] According to the *New York Times*, two of the biggest air ambulance providers are owned by private equity, including KKR.[28] And chances are, your company's HMO plan doesn't cover the $50,000 air ambulance ride, and so you'd likely get stuck with the bill.

But you don't have to ride in on a helicopter to get screwed by private equity. A nonprofit watchdog called the Private Equity Stakeholder Project reported in 2022 that private equity has a habit of contracting with a hospital and then immediately ditching health networks to bill as out-of-network, freeing them up to charge a whole lotta money.[29] But the No Surprises Act would change that and more.

Perhaps the biggest surprise is the bipartisan support for the legislation, despite the big-pocketed opposition. In 2022, Rep. Bobby Scott (D-VA) and Rep. Virginia Foxx (R-NC) co-wrote a love letter for the new law in *The Hill* after a federal district court struck down portions of it. The pair insisted that "threats to this law should not stand."[30] Scott, who has supported raising the minimum wage to $17 per hour, and Foxx, who voted against codifying same-sex marriage, held hands and walked down the Capitol aisle together to protect the law from attempts to weaken it. That's how bipartisan it is.

But this bill was bipartisan from the start. The original co-sponsors, Senators Cassidy and Hassan, agreed that Americans didn't need any more healthcare surprises. Cassidy called it "pro patient," and Hassan said it would "help ensure that Americans aren't left on the hook for these outrageous bills."[31]

Of course, when it comes to healthcare, we can't have nice things float in on a cloud and shoot rainbows at all of us. It's never that simple. ProPublica reported in 2024 that there actually are "some surprises in the No Surprises Act," namely that the law would lead to higher insurance premiums for everyone.[32] It seems that the government had estimated about 17,000 insurance disputes due to the law when the actual number in 2023 was nearly 700,000.[33] Oh, and more than a fifth of insurers failed to pay out awards that year.[34]

Air ambulance groups and healthcare providers meanwhile have filed a few dozen lawsuits, and, as usual, we wind up paying for this. Meanwhile, Envision Healthcare filed for bankruptcy,[35] in part because of "flawed" implementation of the No Surprises Act, wiping out KKR's kajillion-dollar investment. Look at that, somebody was surprised after all.

Not me though. As I've said, the system isn't broken. It's designed to work this way. But all kinds of people—sometimes working as strange bedfellows—continue to work on behalf of all patients and sometimes, they win and so do we.

LIVESTRONG Army

Cancer advocacy wouldn't be where it is today without LIVESTRONG. Period. LIVESTRONG began as the Lance Armstrong Foundation to raise funds for testicular cancer and was rebranded in 2003 shortly before the launch of the organization's ubiquitous yellow wristbands (see Chapter 4), which raised money and awareness for overall cancer advocacy.

But LIVESTRONG was and is more than a cultural firebrand of coolness. They launched LIVESTRONG Day to descend upon Capitol Hill in support of the Cancer Screening, Treatment, and Survivorship Act of 2007,[36] a bipartisan bill designed to help underserved populations get access to cancer screening and care. Armstrong and 200 other cancer survivors from all 50 states helped drum up support for the bill that day in DC. That LIVESTRONG could get the Empire State Building to light up in yellow on the same day was the kind of super cool attention-getting that Lance and his crew could pull off back in the day.[37] I mean, Lance's name went before the Congresspeople's names in headlines about the bill.[38]

Sadly, the bill died for multiple reasons, including the looming 2008 financial crisis and other healthcare legislation competing for lawmakers' attention. But it led the way for the ACA to eventually mandate coverage for preventive services, like screening for breast, colorectal, skin, and cervical cancer.[39]

That's what LIVESTRONG was best at—lending fame and support to draw attention to issues affecting cancer survivors and raising global awareness. Even in a Lance take-down article by *Outside* magazine in 2012, the organization's dedication to survivors was noted: "LIVESTRONG provides an innovative and expanding suite of direct services to help cancer survivors negotiate our Kafkaesque healthcare system."[40]

LIVESTRONG uses its big yellow energy to continue to help cancer patients by funding survivorship programs throughout the country. Their Young Adult Alliance helped advance the cause of young adult cancers (AYA) back when Stupid Cancer was making its way onto the scene, and the LIVESTRONG Foundation funded AYA survivorship studies.[41] As a result, new survivorship models were created, quite possibly affecting your own post-cancer care.[42]

The Academy of Oncology Nurse & Patient Navigators

If there's one piece of advice that I have consistently given to the recently diagnosed, it's that it's important to find an anchor in a sea of chaos. Who better to guide you through rough waters than a trained oncology nurse?

Nearly two decades after Dr. Harold P. Freeman paved the way with the first patient navigation program (see Chapter 5), the oncology nurses came to navigation in full force. Led by oncology nurse and two-time breast cancer survivor Lillie D. Shockney, RN, the Academy of Oncology Nurse & Patient Navigators (AONN) was founded in 2009 to support cancer patients with "professional patient advocates."

What do oncology nurse navigators do? In short, they act as healthcare sherpas, guiding patients through a fragmented and siloed system where you might have three different types of doctors: an oncologist, a radiation oncologist, and a surgeon. They help coordinate care, including screening and procedures, and address barriers like a lack of transportation or childcare, or not being able to speak English. They help patients find doctors, schedule appointments, get financial aid, sign up for clinical trials, and they teach you about your diagnosis and treatments.

Recognizing that cancer has a disproportionate impact on communities of color, people in lower tax brackets, LGBTQ communities, and others, AONN set out to standardize the nurse navigation practice. They focused on a series of standards that includes, among others: qualifications, knowledge, interdisciplinary and interorganizational collaboration, ethics, communication, end of life, advocacy, and survivorship.[43]

The results include faster diagnosis and treatment, encouraging people to stick to their treatment plans, removing barriers to treatment, saving costs from fewer ER visits, providing emotional support, and improving access for underserved communities.[44] Best of all, they normalize support for cancer patients and the people who love them.

Candice Roth, MSN, RN, CENP is the CEO of AONN and a member of We the Patients' Clinical Advisory Council with an oncology nurse background. She told me that patients trust their nurse navigators—often more than other members of their care team—because they're with them through each transition of care, "whether that's chemotherapy, immunotherapy, surgery, radiation, we're there." This kind of support is an "easy sell" to patients. But what about insurers?

"What we are seeing and finding," she said, "and there is some evidence out there to support, is that the navigators are able to keep patients on treatment longer," addressing side effects, reducing no-show rates, and keeping patients out of the hospital, which, of course, saves money for insurers. Helping patients live longer and healthier lives saves costs.

I am so certain that patient advocacy works because I've seen it work. In fact, I would argue that if there is a Mount Rushmore of patient advocacy success, oncology nurse navigation should be chiseled in first.

Breast Cancer Education and Awareness Requires Learning Young (EARLY) Act of 2009

Rep. Debbie Wasserman Schultz (D-FL), a breast cancer survivor and BRCA2 mutation carrier, introduced legislation to raise awareness and support for women aged 45 and younger with breast cancer. Passed in 2010 through the ACA and reauthorized in 2014, the EARLY Act also provided for research into preventing breast cancer in young women.

This may not sound like a big deal, but you have to understand that most breast cancer campaigns are aimed at women over 50 because they're more likely to get diagnosed. But 10 percent of new breast cancer diagnoses are in women forty-five and under.[45] That's one in ten. Picture the quarterback of every football team on an offensive drive having cancer and you get the idea of how prevalent this really is.

"One of the reasons they are diagnosed at a later stage is because many young women don't think they can get breast cancer—that breast cancer is something that only happens to older women," says Wasserman Schultz, whose treatments included a double mastectomy and oophorectomy (removal of the ovaries).[46]

A breast cancer diagnosis when you're young brings additional issues that don't always affect older patients the same way, including fertility during childbearing years. This, I know: If you're a 20-year-old college kid diagnosed with cancer, you're going to have different issues from a 60-year-old with the same diagnosis. In fact, that's why Maimah Karmo of the Tigerlily Foundation also got involved in this initiative. (See Chapter 5.)

The EARLY Act set the stage for the CDC's Bring Your Brave initiative, which used stories of young breast cancer survivors to educate younger women about their risks and options. It also shared preventive screening guidelines with healthcare providers, explaining the breast cancer screening protocols for women with BRCA1 or BRCA2 gene mutations and others who are at a higher risk.

It paved the way for the Protecting Access to Lifesaving Screenings (PALS) Act, which provides insurance coverage for annual mammograms with no co-pays for women starting at age 40 through January 1, 2026.[47] As of this writing, there appears to be no one actively opposing extending this legislation, and lots of cancer and physician organizations have backed it, but they haven't extended funding either. If it dies, insurers might revert to biennial coverage, and that could increase the number of "quarterbacks" as some early detection is missed.

The States That Bought the Ingredients for Obamacare

I have long felt that the entire healthcare industry can make all the money they want—yay, capitalism—just please try to kill us less. To the industry: I'm not here to tell you how to run your business, but can't you profit from *not* harming us, too?

With the ACA on the ropes, it's important to understand that the protections that come with it could get the KO, too. That means we could go back to the pre-Obamacare era when insurance companies could reject an applicant for a health issue, carve out coverage for it, or charge more because of it. Without protections for pre-existing conditions, healthcare insurance could get very expensive for us.

Let's say you've got a bad back and you want health insurance. Well, in a post-ACA world, just like in the pre-ACA world, an insurance company could say, "We'll cover everything except any-thing having to do with your back." It's important to note here that the average price of a common back surgery, lumbar spine fusion, is about $70,000 without insurance.[48]

These protections aren't just for people who get their insurance through the ACA, either. In 2013, before Obamacare kicked in nationwide, nearly one in five applicants were denied coverage in the individual insurance market,[49] often for pre-existing conditions. The ACA wrote protections into federal laws, not just for individual markets, but also for small-group, large-group, and self-insured employer plans. If you're under 65, this likely affects you, unless you're a self-paying Saudi prince or a tech billionaire, I suppose.

When the Trump administration challenged the ACA's consti-tutionality in the US Supreme Court in 2020 while the pandemic raged on, *KFF* looked at what would happen to protections offered by the ACA should it be taken out behind the barn and shot. They explained that protections for people with pre-existing conditions would likely be eliminated because it was baked into the banana bread of Obamacare. "It would be enormously complex to disentan-gle these provisions from the overall healthcare system."[50]

The Health Insurance Portability and Accountability Act of 1996 (HIPAA) offers some protections for people on employer-sponsored group plans, preventing insurance companies from refusing coverage for people with pre-existing conditions. But those "HIPAA conver-sion" policies were so expensive that, says *KFF Health News*, "almost no one could afford them."[51] The same goes for Medicare and Med-icaid. But for the rest of us, hang tight because insurance compa-nies will likely regain the right to protect themselves from the cost of covering the chronically ill and anyone else with a pre-existing condition.[52]

Terrified? Geography might provide a solution, and I don't just mean leaving the United States. There are states that have enacted ACA-style protections, some of them before Obamacare was even a thing and some after the attempts to kill it started. In fact, between early 2018 and late 2019, at least seventeen states jumped on this bandwagon, adopting all or some of the ACA's four core consumer protections, which includes pre-existing conditions.[53]

The old schoolers got on board back in the nineties, including Maine, Massachusetts, New Jersey, New York, and Vermont. All traditionally blue states, but some were under GOP governorships at the time. By the time Obamacare came onto the horizon in the 2010s, six states were "guaranteed issue," meaning that insurers couldn't deny you based on a health issue, so add Washington to that list.[54] These states were all ahead of their time, and their provisions helped pave the way for a national ban on denying coverage for people with pre-existing conditions for most kinds of insurance coverage, via the ACA law.

It worked in theory more than in reality.

Kentucky also implemented some protections shortly after the Clinton Obamacare-esque plan flopped in the nineties, but it didn't last long. By the end of the decade, numerous insurance carriers withdrew from the state's health insurance market,[55] and prices rose. Then in 2000, Kentucky repealed the guaranteed issue protections and created a high-risk pool[56] with often costly plans that cover "expensive" patients. As AP noted, Governor Brereton C. Jones "envisioned a system in which coverage would be accessible and affordable for everyone in the state, regardless of health history. Instead, dozens of insurers bailed out of Kentucky, and costs for individual coverage soared."[57]

New Hampshire had a similar problem and ended guaranteed issue in the individual market in 2002 after dozens of insurance companies left the state and established a high-risk pool that subsidized coverage for the sickest of the sick.[58] Washington also scaled back some of its insurance offerings before Obamacare went into effect in 2014.

These provisions weren't perfect in their implementation, but they did set a precedent that hey, maybe we shouldn't penalize people for getting sick, no matter where they get their insurance? As KFF reported, "Some higher-cost health conditions, like cancer, diabetes, or even pregnancy, left people trying to buy their own health coverage 'uninsurable' before the Affordable Care Act." That's because the 5 percent of people with the highest healthcare costs are responsible for half of total healthcare spending.[59] Without ACA protections, insurance companies will see us coming and think, *That's gonna hurt.* Only, without the ACA's protections, they can more readily avoid the pain.

Before Obamacare, individual market insurers in all but the OG five states with guaranteed issue protections could deny coverage for cancer survivors and decline medications, including chemo.[60] They could even deny coverage for certain occupations, such as firefighters, meat packers, pilots, and professional athletes. People like me who were born with a (pricey to care for) congenital disease could also be denied coverage in the individual market in most states, forever tying us to jobs where the health insurance is adequate, as though only employees of medium-to-large corporations are worthy of decent healthcare.

So, will state-level protections for pre-existing conditions be able to survive if Obamacare doesn't? John E. McDonough, DrPH, MPA, a Harvard University TH Chan School for Public Health professor, provided the answer back in 2018: "The real-world difficulty with guaranteed issue is that, absent an individual mandate to purchase health insurance, the policy by itself will trigger substantial health insurance premium increases."[61]

Okay, but the OG states thought of that already, many issuing state-level individual mandates that impose a penalty for not carrying health insurance. The truth is that without the ACA's federal subsidies, individual market insurance will likely get really expensive, pricing people out, like we saw in early 2026, likely leaving just wealthy and very sick people, who might get help in high-risk pools, on the rolls.

And yet.

Guaranteed issue is super popular in a bipartisan way. Americans like it no matter how they feel about Obamacare. As our Harvard professor McDonough said, "No provision in any of the ACA repeal bills instigated more anger and fury among the public than the Republican assaults on guaranteed issue. And rejection of this proposal was not confined to the general public. Indeed, almost all health sector stakeholders roundly rejected the idea, including hospitals, physicians, labor unions, consumers, and, yes, even insurance companies."[62]

It became part of the conversation thanks to five states that implemented protections at the state level thirty years ago, when Obamacare was just a gleam in Nancy Pelosi's eye. No matter what happens to the ACA, America, for the most part, wants to protect people who have pre-existing conditions from being discriminated against in their health insurance plans. Somewhere, somebody is working on ways to preserve that protection, no matter which state you live in.

Assorted Protections

Behind the scenes, all sorts of people have been working to provide "healthcare consumers" with protections. When the protections get taken away at the federal level, they tend to pop up at the state level and vice versa, like a game of medical Whac-a-mole™. Here are some of the protections that have come and gone and sometimes, come again:

The Credit Report Relief Rule

Before the Biden administration left office in January 2025, the Consumer Financial Protection Bureau (CFPB) finalized a rule that banned the inclusion of medical bills on credit reports. It's not like cancer patients go out and blow it all on chemo like they're buying Escalades and Cristal to impress their friends, right? This isn't about financial irresponsibility. It's about how America's healthcare system is designed like the classic game Operation, where one wrong move can set off the buzzer.

But it didn't last long. By July of that year, a federal judge in Texas, appointed by Trump, overruled it, saying it exceeded the CFPB's authority. Too bad, because removing medical debt from credit reports was expected to make credit scores for many people rise about 20 points.[63]

The states to the rescue! Or some of them. Fifteen states have removed many medical bills from credit reports, and it's mostly blue states and the usual suspects: California, Colorado, Connecticut, Delaware, Illinois, Maine, Maryland, Minnesota, New Jersey, New York, Oregon, Rhode Island, Virginia, Vermont, and Washington.[64]

In these states, anyhow, medical debt won't sink your credit when you look for a place to live or work or a car to drive—at least for now.

Hospital Price Transparency

For a long time, hospitals kept their price lists, called "chargemasters," a secret. If you got a test or procedure at a hospital, how much it cost would depend on your insurance plan. *The New York Times* showed just how different the costs to you could be, with the price tag of a colonoscopy at one hospital ranging from $782 to $2,144 depending on the plan. They didn't want you to know until your bill came in. Reports the *Times*, "This secrecy has allowed hospitals to tell patients that they are getting 'steep' discounts, while still charging them many times what a public program like Medicare is willing to pay."[65]

The idea of hospital price transparency initially got some traction during President Trump's first term in office, when he issued an executive order in 2019 requiring most health insurers to tell patients what their hospital procedures and tests will cost.[66] Then in 2021, President Biden doubled-down, requiring hospitals to publish price data.[67] But that wasn't as helpful as some wished it would be, in part because of limited enforcement.[68] The editorial board of one medical journal was unimpressed with what they called "hospital-centric" price transparency, explaining, "Patient-centric price transparency is required; sadly, it seems that hospitals will not provide these data without tighter regulation."[69]

The patient rights group Power to the Patients reported in late 2024 that less than 40 percent of hospitals were compliant with transparency measures. Their spokesperson, the rapper Fat Joe, told *People* that, "Our very own healthcare system is robbing all of us. We just need the prices."[70]

So, Trump hunkered down in February 2025 through an executive order with a title that would never fit on a marquee: "Making America Healthy Again by Empowering Patients with Clear, Accurate, and Actionable Healthcare Pricing Information." Essentially, it claimed that hospitals hadn't been held accountable by "Sleepy Joe," but don't worry, they would be now. As Louisiana Senator John Kennedy, tweeted, "If Louisianians can find the price of a side of mashed potatoes at any of the 600 Cracker Barrel locations around the country, they ought to be able to find the price of a blood test at the nearest hospital, too."[71]

Or bagels in New York, crab cakes in Maryland, steaks in Omaha, TexMex everywhere. Hospital price transparency is popular nationwide, with 96 percent of Americans in support, says PatientRightsAdvocate.org, and politicians on both sides of the political aisle support it.[72]

Charity Care for Medical Debt

Only a third of people who qualify for charity care actually receive it, according to research by Dollar For, the nonprofit that helps patients apply for financial assistance from the hospital that I profiled in Chapter 6. Their website explains, "Every year, patients are billed $14 billion that should be waived through hospital financial assistance."[73]

While most hospitals are required to discount or forgive bills for qualified patients, "they don't make it easy," explains Dollar For. *The Wall Street Journal* reports that nonprofit hospitals take an estimated

$60 billion in tax breaks each year in exchange for offering financial assistance programs for needy patients. But they "put up obstacles, delay checking eligibility, and sometimes press for payments that aren't refunded."[74] Not only that, but more than half of eligible patients never even learn about these programs.[75] Dollar For has eliminated more than $100 million in medical debt for thousands of patients nationwide.[76]

As a new oncology nurse, Christy Snodgrass noticed the massive amounts of debt her hospital patients often took on. She left the bedside for advocacy to bring transparency and reform to the US healthcare system. She told me, "One of the things that pushed me in the direction that I am in now is that my cancer patients were drowning in medical debt." In 2025, she testified on behalf of Dollar For at the Texas State Capitol in Austin about proposed legislation that would require nonprofit hospitals to automatically screen patients for charity care assistance,[77] explaining that hospitals are required to have the programs but not to actually apply patients for them.[78]

"I see that healthcare is on the brink," she told me. "No matter what end of the political spectrum that you're on agrees that there needs to be change."

KFF estimates about 40 percent of Americans carry some sort of medical or dental debt.[79] Sometimes it's those lab tests your doctor ran before you've hit your annual deductible or a dental bill when you don't have insurance for your teeth. A *KFF Health* survey found that half of adults with healthcare debt owe less than $2,500, while 12 percent owe more than $10,000 (Figure 7.1).[80] And it affects people of all income levels, except maybe the billionaires.

Meanwhile, the National Consumer Law Center has written the Model Medical Debt Protection Act. It's not a federal bill, but a set of guidelines for states to adopt to improve financial assistance policies in hospitals and assist patients who qualify "to reduce burdensome medical debt and to protect patients in their dealings with medical creditors, medical debt buyers, and medical debt collectors with respect to such debt."[81]

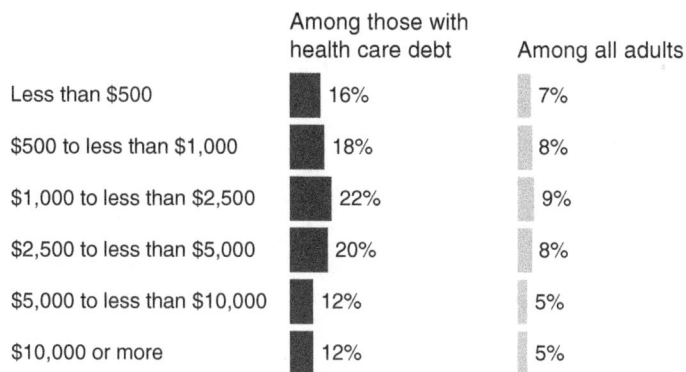

	Among those with health care debt	Among all adults
Less than $500	16%	7%
$500 to less than $1,000	18%	8%
$1,000 to less than $2,500	22%	9%
$2,500 to less than $5,000	20%	8%
$5,000 to less than $10,000	12%	5%
$10,000 or more	12%	5%

FIGURE 7.1 About Half of Adults with Health Care Debt Owe Less Than $2,500.
Source: KFF Health Care Debt Survey (Feb. 25–Mar. 20, 2022)

Meanwhile, a handful of states already mandate discounts for low-income patients under certain criteria, including California, Connecticut, Illinois, Maine, Maryland, Nevada, New Jersey, New York, Rhode Island, and Washington.[82]

Universal Healthcare for Oregon

No, this isn't a *Portlandia* sketch. Since the 2010s, Oregon has been working toward actual "quality, affordable, universal, single-payer healthcare"[83] for their citizens. It would mean that people would keep their healthcare coverage even if they lost their jobs, eliminate co-pays and deductibles, reduce administrative costs, and simplify billing, among other seemingly utopian goodies.[84]

They've passed a series of legislation, including an act that "prevents debt collectors from wiping out someone's entire bank account by protecting the first $2,500" and a law designed to protect pharmacies and patients from the effects of unregulated pharmacy benefits managers (PBMs).[85]

Much of the work lies ahead of them, and Health Care for All Oregon expects to bring it to the ballot in 2027 or 2028 with a roll-out estimated for 2030.[86]

Oregon isn't the first state to try to implement universal healthcare. Vermont, home of Senator Bernie "healthcare is a human right" Sanders, was the first state to vote for a publicly financed healthcare system back in 2014, only to abandon their plans when Governor Peter Shumlin pulled the plug over its costs, insisting it simply wasn't the right time for it.[87]

California, too, backed off their universal healthcare plan in 2022 when Governor Gavin "We believe in the right to quality health care" Newsom and other Democratic lawmakers shied away from introducing legislation. Colorado's related 2016 ballot initiative failed, thanks to healthcare industry opposition, and Washington's Senate and House bills both died in committee in 2025.[88]

All states have an uphill battle, because they'd need federal money from Medicare and Medicaid to cover the cost, first securing a waiver to apply via the Department of Health and Human Services, which, you may have noticed, has been in a bit of disarray.

"States are required to balance their budget every year," writes Tobias Coughlin-Bogue in the progressive Seattle newspaper *The Stranger,* "and if they've suddenly taken on the cost of covering all residents while losing a major revenue source earmarked for that purpose, they won't be able to balance shit."[89]

Arkansas PBM Law

Meanwhile in Arkansas, Governor Sarah Huckabee Sanders signed legislation in early 2025 to ban PBMs from owning pharmacies, the first law of its kind nationwide. In other words, the middlemen taking a piece of the pharmacy action can't also own the pharmacy.

Arkansas State Senator Kim Hammer said, "This legislation addresses what has become a blatant monopolization of pharmacy reimbursements by PBMs that control 80 percent of the market."

MedPage said the Arkansas law is no magical solution, "but it is a good first step and a signal that states are no longer waiting for Congress to untangle the complexities of prescription drug pricing."[90]

In all, twenty-four states passed thirty-three bills regulating PBMs in 2024. Idaho and Vermont banned spread pricing, when PBMs reimburse pharmacies at a lower rate than the money they received from insurers. Other states passed laws requiring PBMs to report the rebates they received, while still others worked to legislate PBM reform.[91]

Pharmacist called 2025 the "Year of PBM Reform," unifying the pharmacy profession. "From coast to coast, states are passing legislation that increases transparency, protects patient access, and ensures pharmacies are paid fairly for the medications and services they provide." And that's good for pharmacies and patients alike.[92]

We the Rabblerousers

More often than not, your healthcare is not up for your vote. State and federal lawmakers do the voting on things that matter for your health, which is why it's so important to cast your vote for the people who will represent your best interests wisely. But the things they vote on start with people just like you who introduce ideas, rally support, battle attacks on their healthcare rights, organize patients and healthcare workers, write legislation, lobby lawmakers, write op-eds, spread the news on social media, and make things happen.

And they—you—are relentless.

8 We the Organized

To determine what's next for cancer advocacy, we need to look at Detroit six decades ago. That's when President Lyndon Johnson signed into law the National Traffic and Motor Vehicle Safety Act, in 1966, back when seatbelts were considered a luxury item, like heated seats or Corinthian leather upholstery. In those days, US automakers were largely unregulated and car safety was an afterthought.

But then Ralph Nader pulled up. The consumer advocate's best-selling takedown of the auto industry, *Unsafe at Any Speed*, led to the first significant car safety legislation in America.[1] This was the OG Nader, taking on the Chevrolet Corvair and therefore Detroit giant General Motors, calling their hot new sports car a "one-car accident" for its tendency to roll over.[2]

Before Nader, the industry's million car accidents with 40,000 fatalities, 110,000 permanent disabilities, and 1.5 million injuries in the United States per year were largely chalked up to driver error and bad roads.[3] But the Corvair's short rollover history made it the perfect poster car for the lack of focus on safety in the automobile industry at the time. Nader said, "It was stylistic pornography over engineering integrity," and by 1969, the Corvair[i] was discontinued.[4]

Thanks to the new law, supported in part by the American Automobile Association, the federal government now had the authority to set and enforce minimum safety standards for all new cars sold in the United States. We didn't just get seatbelts. In time, we also got shatter-resistant windshields, antilock brakes, automobile recalls, and the first crash test dummy taking the hit for us, and in GM cars no less. And the industry won, too, in lawsuits never filed, as seatbelt use reduced the fatality and serious injury rate over time by up to 75 percent in crashes.[5]

What does this have to do with healthcare? It illustrates how consumer protection advocacy works. Look at it as if it were a cake. The recipe would go like this:

- 1 cup of statistics on harm or potential harm to consumers
- 1 cup of relentless advocacy, preferably by a high-profile celebrity or expert
- 1 cup of publicity (book, media coverage, social media exposure)
- ½ cup of consumer storytelling ("This bad thing happened to me because of this product.")
- ½ cup of Congressional support (bill sponsorship and votes)
- ¼ cup of measurable support from a major nonprofit or not-for-profit national member association (funding, bill drafting or amicus briefs, publicity, membership support)
- ¼ cup health economic cost benefit
- 1 tsp. of carefully directed shame

In cancer advocacy's cake, we need to be more like OG Nader and bring the right ingredients. Until now, we've thought of cancer patients as victims of a system that predetermines your outcome

---

[i]Guess whose dad was driving a Corvair at the time.

for you, depending on your insurance coverage, geography, and demographics, when really, what we are is a millions-strong group of healthcare consumers. It's a for-profit market with shareholders and quarterly reports, and we are their consumers. Consumers in a mall that we never wanted to shop in because no one plans to get sick, but consumers nevertheless. And like all consumers, we need protections from an industry designed to make profits.

In most nonprofits, running defense, plugging holes, and triaging is the modus operandi, but these can be Band-Aids. They're working on behalf of the patient, but no one's fighting for the healthcare consumer. Cancer advocacy is still based on the nonprofit old school of thought: the green ribbons, yellow wristbands, and pink stand mixers that sprung up in the nineties and 2000s. That's when there was no social media, save for Myspace maybe, and good IRL social protests raised tons of money. Nonprofits kept popping up whenever somebody got cancer and didn't want anyone else to go through the same ordeal. I mean, it's easy to get 501(3)(c) tax status, so why not form a nonprofit for [insert cancer type here]? It's grief nonprofitism, and it's reactionary.

Yes, I know I just described exactly what I did with Stupid Cancer in 2007. Guilty as charged. But I did it with a degree of conscious ignorance, incubated and curated by some of the best nonprofit leaders out there. It was a mistake that went right, fueled in large part by my relentless drive to make cancer suck less for people who aren't geriatric or pediatric and to introduce the idea that quality of life is as important as quality of care. We had to explain that we wanted to help people *today*, not "one day," and not everyone understood. But enough did.

I never set out to run a nonprofit and I didn't know what the hell I was doing. But I knew how to build a brand, and I understood the concept of a nonprofit as a business, not a side hustle to the founder's "real" job. Yet I hated the idea of begging for money. To me, it felt like standing on the corner with an organ grinder monkey on your shoulder.

The entire fundraising-palooza can get in the way of a nonprofit's true mission because of the way it's set up. Nonprofit leader Vu Le of Nonprofit AF has publicly called out some of the "crappy practices" that funders force nonprofits to go through to secure cash, including "a five-page narrative, eight attachments, and . . . a blood oath to give up their firstborn, for a $1,000 grant."[6] It's funny/not funny, and it's indicative of the hoops that nonprofits have to jump through to secure funding.

Donors want a report of the quantitative impact of their money, and they want their donations to go directly to the mission, not the infrastructure that holds it all up. But if nonprofits don't have electricity, employees, payroll, and health benefits, there is no mission. Think about it: If your nonprofit has a billion-dollar budget, don't you want a leader who can run a billion-dollar company? That kind of talent needs to be compensated—not in crazy tech CEO numbers, but in realistic salaries for the extent of the job.

The founder and President of the Charity Defense Council and one of the most influential human beings of my career, Dan Pallotta, argues that it takes money to make money—even in nonprofits. The author of *The Everyday Philanthropist* and the TEDx speaker of "The Way We Think about Charity is Dead Wrong," Dan is a rabblerouser in the nonprofit space. On my *Out of Patients* podcast, he said, "Most nonprofits are still driven by their fear of keeping overhead low." That's because, Dan said, "You can go ahead and ask a hundred people on the street, 'How do you decide which charity to give to?' And they'll say the ones with the lowest overhead and don't pay their CEOs very much." But here's the rub: "A nonprofit that keeps its overhead low and keeps its salaries low is not the nonprofit that's going to change the world."[7]

That's mostly the small, scrappy nonprofits, the sub-$5 million, Sisyphean types. Yet quite a few of the patient advocate nonprofits are seventy-year-old, billion-dollar, massive organizations with names everyone knows, and they're good at doing what they've always done: raising awareness and money. But like a ginormous aircraft carrier, they're not quick to pivot.

Together, these two groups make up Nonprofit Patient Advocacy 1.0. It's like Web 1.0, the read-only version of the internet written in HTML and used primarily as reference, when what cancer advocacy needs now is the 2.0 version, which is interactive and proactive.

Stupid Cancer was a directory of resources, fully 1.0 when I launched it, and it needed to be. But I funded it differently than the usual nonprofit. I secured commercial dollars as a nonprofit to produce content on my internet radio show that was evergreen, non-branded, and unscripted. And I got lucky, because this new internet thing was coming along, and so I was able to start creating revenue to at least get my nonprofit off the ground, pay an intern, build the website, and do all the little things a startup needs to do.

It made sense for the times as it did for all cancer advocacy non-profits: Give us money so we can help people with cancer. A lot of good has come from it through many cancer advocacy nonprofits of varying sizes, including money for research, legal resources, education, and support, not to mention cool T-shirts and a sense of community.

But there's no real forecasting in nonprofit patient advocacy, not as it stands today. They're just waiting for more people to get sick and need their services. They're mechanically driven, not marketing engines for populist movements to affect change through consumer protections. They're not set up to prevent buffoonery in healthcare, only to mitigate it.

If it sounds like I'm queuing up an argument for treating advocacy like a business, there are downfalls there, too. Private equity might be brilliant at spotting shiny opportunities like novel therapies, diagnostics, and AI wizardry. But they so often fail to ask the patients they're designed to help, "Does this work for you?" They invest millions in the Next Big Thing, only to watch it stumble because they forgot the advocacy part.

But ignoring advocacy isn't just shortsighted, it's downright stupid. Take clinical trials, for instance. When you bring patients into the fold early, they run more smoothly. Enrollment is faster, retention skyrockets, and outcomes improve.

But even then, advocacy isn't just about trials and approvals. It's about the whole messy, terrifying, beautiful journey of being a patient who never signed up for the role. Cancer advocacy matters, but how it's delivered needs to change. Most nonprofits and plenty of private equity firms tend to focus on just one circle in the patient advocacy Venn diagram (Figure 8.1).

- **Support:** This involves triaging cancer patients with the support they need to face the consequences of practical issues, like paying for fertility treatments, addressing lifestyle issues, hosting meet-ups, and providing information so that cancer sucks less.
- **Research:** I don't just mean medical research. I mean research into survivorship, best practices, standards of care, patient navigation, and other quality of life issues.

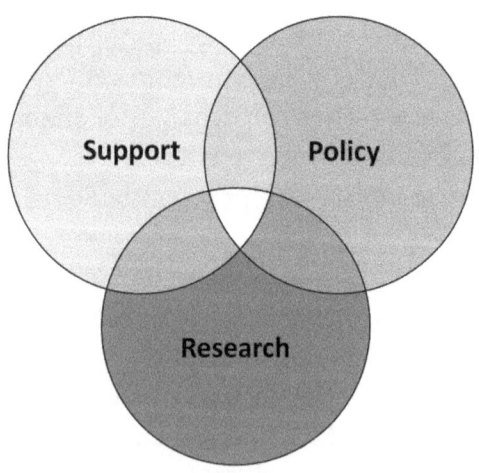

FIGURE 8.1 Patient Advocacy: A Venn Diagram

- **Policy:** These are the nuts and bolts of healthcare rules, guidelines, and laws that I've highlighted throughout the book, such as the hospital billing transparency laws, mammogram guidelines, survivorship standards, and mother of them all, the ACA.

Nobody needs to do all three parts, but that sweet spot where the Venn diagram overlaps is where the patient advocacy revolution will be sparked. And it's already starting to be televised, or at least, posted on Instagram. The doctors sharing stories of how insurance companies have impeded their ability to practice medicine. The patients reporting prior-authorization denials. The #freeluigi hashtags. The surprising bipartisan support for PBM reform.

In this post-CDC bloodbath era, where the people in charge of ensuring Americans' access to healthcare chose to cut off the only coordinated research program in this country focused on saving kids with brain cancer,[8] we must move to the 2.0 phase, beyond the knee jerk, "cancer nearly killed me," reactionary, bereavement stage. We must instead be proactive, where we forecast instead of react, because the rules of the game have changed. To borrow a line from Wayne Gretzky, it's time for us to skate to where the puck is going.

Wall Street rewards revenue, not survival, and Wall Street runs our for-profit healthcare system. We used to be able to count on federal agencies to have our backs as patients and advocates, but if President Trump's second administration is any indication, that's gone. At least, for now. All you have to do is flip open a news app and read:

- *The Guardian:* "More patients may die as a result of plans drawn up by the Trump administration to cut billions of dollars from the National Cancer Institute (NCI), veteran federal government workers and experts have warned."[9]
- *The Associated Press:* "The cuts threaten to derail scores of clinical trials of new treatments, with universities saying they'll have to "stop or not enroll patients.""

- "Let's think about that. 'A clinical trial is a last hope for a lot of people,' [attorney representing the plaintiffs, John] Bueker said."[10]
- *19th News:* "Health and Human Services Secretary Robert F. Kennedy Jr. this week defunded research in messenger RNA vaccines, which could create a chilling effect that could jeopardize efforts to develop vaccines against breast cancer, experts said."[11]
- *STAT News:* "These cuts would be felt in every corner of oncology—research, safety-net programs, innovation, and, most painfully, our patients."
- "There are obvious effects of slashing budgets. Research funding cuts will mean fewer federal trials, slower drug development, and slower progress toward fighting and curing cancer."[12]
- *WHYY:* "Efforts to find better and new treatments for cancer has, for the most part, been a universally supported endeavor," [William] Sherman [of the American Cancer Society's Cancer Action Network] said, "a nonpartisan issue."

"Until now."

"'I've never met an elected official who tells me no to my face,' Sherman said, referring to gathering support in Washington, DC for research efforts. 'But we know by their voting behaviors that not everybody is with us right now. And they need to be.'"[13]

The King of the World

Like Medicare and Medicaid in the 1960s and the ACA in the 2010s, we need to add and reinstate consumer protections for patients, especially now that these programs have been hit and steerage is filling up with ocean water. But nonprofits—the 1.0 versions—typically aren't set up to provide protections. They can increase awareness that the boat's sinking and raise funds for one day patching up the hull and someday building impact-resistant boats, but they're not designed to watch for icebergs in the first place and steer the whole damn thing around them. And these days, there are icebergs *everywhere*.

Take, for instance, the ransom note that UnitedHealthcare wrote to patients after Wall Street became dissatisfied with their margins, with profits dipping from $15.8 billion in 2024 to $14.3 billion post-Luigi. They announced that they would raise premiums by double digits, slash benefits, purge more than a half-million members, and cut providers out of networks. All so that shareholders can sleep better at night.

The worst part is how normalized this all feels. A company with $84 billion in Medicare Advantage overpayments still cries poverty. Congress shrugs. Employers pass costs to workers. Doctors drown in paperwork while the umbrella healthcare conglomerate United-Health Group becomes the largest employer of doctors in the country. Meanwhile, patients, the ones supposedly "valued," get fewer options and higher bills every single year.

This is the cycle. Squeeze patients until they skip care. They get sicker. They hit the ER. Costs spike. Wall Street panics. Lather, rinse, repeat. The only "value-based care" happening here is value for investors.

For every $100 a healthcare consumer spends, $16 goes to the insurance company.[14] Accounting for administrative costs, both in health insurance and by hospitals, only $68 goes toward actual care.[15] The shareholders, however, make out nicely. As the *Pennsylvania Capital-Star* reported shortly after the murder of United-Healthcare CEO Brian Thompson: *"Think of it this way: A person who owned a single $500 share of UnitedHealth Group stock at the start of the year would get rewarded, at the year's end, with $7.29 of America's healthcare spending, despite contributing precisely nothing to American healthcare."*[16]

In the months after the murder, UnitedHealthcare's stock plummeted and then, Warren Buffett scooped it out of the bargain bin, snatching up about 5 million shares for roughly $1.6 billion,[17] and other investors followed suit. Eight months after the deadly incident, the company's stock had "its best day in years," says *Barron's*,[18] outperforming the S&P 500.[19] As of this writing, the stock has a "buy" rating, meaning analysts expect it to outperform the market over the next 12 months.[20] Maybe that's because their chief financial officer promised to "get back to the swagger the company once had."[21]

Unfortunately, Big Insurance cannot be shamed into doing the right thing. They are the direct result of President Nixon's HMO Act of 1973 (see Chapter 1)—the slag, the impurities in the smelting process of healthcare. The only way to hit them where it hurts is to affect their bottom line, like the infamous GameStop short, when a ragtag gang of Redditors drove up the video game store's stock prices, forcing Wall Street-types to dump their holdings at a loss. But that would be just a stunt, and a $1.6 trillion industry[22] like health insurance would feel the effects only briefly. The math works in their favor to make the money back.

Consider healthcare whistleblower and former Cigna Vice President Wendell Potter's observation that UnitedHealthcare is no longer just a healthcare company, but a "vertically integrated empire that controls doctors, clinics, the pharmacy supply chain, data, and payments. It touches nearly every part of care delivery in this country."[23] Maybe it's too big to fail?

Meanwhile, the Congressional Budget Office (CBO) has their own predictions of the effects of the OBBB:

- 7.8 million more uninsured from Medicaid changes
- 3.1 million more uninsured from changes to the ACA
- 900,000 more uninsured because of the rule changes to the ACA, such as a shortened open enrollment period and the addition of required documentation
- 4.2 million more uninsured from the expiration of enhanced premium tax credits[24]

No wonder Senate Democratic Leader Chuck Schumer (D-NY) called the bill, now a law, the "We're All Going to Die" Act. Weeks before it passed, he spoke on the Senate floor, explaining, "The CBO just announced their bill will kick millions more people off their healthcare than we originally thought, not only by attacking

Medicaid, but by crippling the ACA, private insurance, and even Medicare, now."

Yes, Medi*care*. Thanks to the bill, prior authorizations have weaseled their way into a six-state pilot program in Medicare Advantage that uses AI to determine whether Grandpa will get knee arthroscopy or incontinence treatment, for instance, or if a robot has determined it's not medically necessary because it's "wasteful care."[25]

The New York Times explained, "But while experts agree that wasteful spending exists, they worry that the pilot program may pave the way for traditional Medicare to adopt some of the most unpopular practices of private insurers."[26]

To quote the classic 1979 movie *When a Stranger Calls*, "It's coming from inside the house."

Us Versus Them

The healthcare system is rigged against us. It's time we rig it against them. The Nonprofit 2.0 model shifts the frame from charity for victims to rights for consumers and power for patients. The ACA gave us a taste of that with protections around pre-existing conditions, preventive screenings, and appeals. But the ACA was built around preserving industry profits, a compromise that looked like we took a step closer to universal healthcare, when in reality, patients got some protections, but the insurers still controlled the system. Now, Big Insurance makes more money by delaying or denying care than by covering it, and AI is making it easier and faster to boost their bottom line.

Why do we tolerate it? Would we accept a car that got worse every year—a "one-car accident"—but costs twice as much? Or a phone with fewer features every time you upgrade? Health insurance is the one product in America that reliably gets worse while becoming unaffordable to own. There's no alternative market and we all need health insurance.

Nonprofit 1.0 has defined the last few decades of cancer advocacy. These groups step in once patients are already in crisis. They provide much-needed money, navigation, fertility help, peer groups, and mental health support. But it's triage. It helps, but it doesn't change the conditions that caused the crisis in the first place. It's the Support circle of our Venn diagram.

Yet there's hope. For instance, we've finally started fighting back against the Pharmacy Benefits Manager (PBM) racket (see Chapter 7), one of the most abusive, opaque, and damaging pieces of the healthcare system, and we've done it in a bipartisan way.

Meanwhile, North Carolina's "Care First Act" set out to lower healthcare costs and increase price transparency by taking a long overdue swipe at prior auths. One of the bill's authors, who is also a physician, Rep. Grans Campbell, told a local radio station, "The parade of people that are trying to interfere with the relationship of the patient and their physician has got to stop, and this is one of the great first steps to do that."[27]

The thing about state-level legislation is that when it passes in one state, other states jump on it, introducing their own bills, and sometimes, that success finds its way into the federal level, like a metastasis, only for good. North Carolina's prior auth law, which my friend Sally Neely Nix calls a "test kitchen" for federal legislation, led to or at least rode alongside a wave of related state-level healthcare consumer protection bills in California, Colorado, Indiana, Iowa, Montana, and Virginia. Maryland passed a law regulating AI in insurance denials, and other states have gotten on board proposing and, in some cases, passing similar legislation, including Arizona, Connecticut, Massachusetts, North Dakota, Pennsylvania, and Texas.

Florida also fought for mandatory human review of insurance claim denials, but it died in committee, and though that's disappointing, for a state that's working to make polio great again, this was a welcomed attempt to protect patients in a place that's not exactly known for it. What's important is that all of these states are not just red or blue, Republican- or Democrat-leaning, and yet they can all get behind one thing: protecting healthcare consumers.

State-level, bi-partisan pushback can and has led to federal reforms. Remember how guaranteed issue and community rating, which protected patients with pre-existing conditions when buying health insurance, started thirty years ago in states like Kentucky and New Jersey? (See Chapter 7.) You can see them in the ACA.

It was "Romneycare," Massachusetts' precursor to Obamacare, that introduced the individual mandate, requiring all citizens to have healthcare coverage. The ACA's Medicaid expansion waivers were tested out in Arizona, Oregon, and Tennessee first. The No Surprises Act's hospital pricing transparency law got its start at the state level, and insulin price caps had their origins in Colorado before passing in multiple states, but they didn't make it past Congressional committees at the federal level. This time, anyhow.

Working Around the Workarounds

For every new protection we manage to wrestle from the system, the industry tries to find a way around it, and that workaround often makes them gobs of money. The ACA's medical loss ratio (MLR) provision is one of those protections, a metric for the percentage of your healthcare that goes toward claims and services instead of administrative costs and profit. It forces insurance companies to allot at least 80 percent of the money that comes in on actual care and all the things any reasonable patient would think their premiums, copays, and deductibles pay for.

Naturally, Big Insurance found a way around it. How? Insurers are bound by the MLR, but "healthcare delivery" is not. As a result, insurance companies like Cigna and UnitedHealthcare began buying up physician practices and clinics and then pointing their insurance enrollees toward their own doctors.

"They're making money hand over fist by self-dealing," whistle-blower Wendell Potter told me. The author of the bestselling book *Deadly Spin*, Wendell got a standing ovation after his keynote speech at Stupid Cancer's 2012 OMG! Cancer Summit for Young Adults, and I witnessed the Wendell-mania first-hand. Wendell knows his shit, and he often shares his insights and warnings with Congress through testimony and with readers through his *HEALTH CARE uncovered* Substack.

"I saw how they confuse their customers and dump the sick—all so they can satisfy their Wall Street investors."[28] Wendell left the Dark Side, but he didn't go into hiding and he couldn't just stay quiet, not with Obamacare, the first significant healthcare reform since the Clintons, on the table, and the usual suspects crying "Socialism!"

He'd seen first-hand the effects of our fractured healthcare system when he visited a pop-up clinic at a fairground in Wise County, Tennessee, where hundreds of uninsured people showed up for medical and dental care they couldn't otherwise afford. To him, it looked like a movie set or a war zone, and he was forever changed by what he'd seen.

He went on to help mitigate the industry's spin because he knew what they would say. Though the ACA was a major step forward for so many healthcare consumers, it was never the end-all, be-all of healthcare magic, waving a magic wand over us all. Wendell called it a "pit stop" in a never-ending battle that shows just how good corporate America is at getting what it wants.[29] The MLR provision is a solid example of the effects of healthcare legislation opening the doors for even more mendacity.

"I wouldn't say that we're close to the finish line by any means, but we're getting people to understand the shortcomings of even the Affordable Care Act," he wrote, "and how that well-intentioned provision has incentivized insurance companies to do what they've been doing in recent years."

But it isn't just the ACA that's been plagued by workarounds. Medicare Advantage, which Wendell calls, "neither Medicare nor an advantage" and a "money-making scam,"[30] allows private insurance companies to administer health benefits, mostly through HMOs or PPOs to Medicare enrollees who opt in. It comes from the Medicare Modernization Act passed under President Bush in 2003. The "advantage" part is supposed to provide enrollees with added benefits such as lower or no cost premiums and additional coverage for dental and vision care. But audits have found that they provided yet another way for health insurers to stick their hands in the cookie jar.

The Wall Street Journal reported in 2024 that several insurers bilked the U.S. government, and therefore taxpayers, of $50 billion for diseases that were never treated. Here's the scam: Insurers practice "diagnostic upcoding" by adding diagnoses in medical charts, sometimes using AI, for diseases that patients hadn't been treated for.[31] Kaiser Permanente even offered doctors bottles of champagne and cash bonuses for adding diagnoses.[32] Several insurers overbilled the government, on average upwards of $1,000 per patient.[33] *The New York Times* reported that eight of the ten biggest Medicare Advantage insurers—familiar names like Humana, CVS Health, Blue Cross/Blue Shield, and Cigna—have submitted inflated bills.[34]

It has been so lucrative that nearly three-quarters of United-Healthcare's 2021 revenues came from Medicare Advantage, Wendell reports.[35] In 2025, Medicare Advantage cost the government an estimated $84 billion more than original flavor Medicare in overpayments, mainly from two practices: favorable selection and coding intensity. According to *Healthcare Brew*, Medicare Advantage experiences favorable selection when the (mostly) healthier people who choose the plan because it's cheaper don't actually use it, but their insurers still bill the government the negotiated set rate and keep the difference.[36]

"Coding intensity" is the lingo to describe the upcoding of Medicare Advantage medical records, a practice not possible in the original fee-for service arrangement (which, by the way, *Healthcare Brew* abbreviates as FFS, as in, "For fuck's sake, don't sign up for Medicare Advantage," I guess).

If you think you're immune to all these shenanigans because your health plan comes from your employer, not the government, think again. Wendell told me that employees are "being fleeced day in and day out without realizing it." That's because for most employer health plans, the employer is the insurer. The insurance company merely administers the benefits, putting the risk entirely on the employer. But they do that while keeping employers uninformed about negotiations with hospitals and physician practices.

This matters, especially now, because employers are covering upwards of 80 percent of healthcare premiums for single employees and 68 percent for families and yet, says New City Insurance, "they're often left in the dark about where that money actually goes."[37]

Wendell says that when he worked in healthcare, part of his job was to pin the blame for high insurance costs on everyone but insurers, including "greedy" doctors, drug and medical device companies, and hospitals. Oh, and we the patients. "Also among the guilty, I'd hasten to add, were regular folks who go to the doctor too much and overuse the healthcare system."[38]

"Overuse?" How can you overuse something that's saving your life? No wonder *KFF Health News* called GoFundMe a medical care "utility." The number of medical funding crowdsourcing accounts increased 25 times between 2001 and 2020.[39] Too many of us are going into debt just to get healthcare because the system is rigged against us. It sets its own prices, pushes costs onto consumers, avoids paying for treatments, lines its own pockets while we pay the price—some of us with our lives.

It's time we build on Nonprofit 1.0's focus on defensive triage, which works like an ER, to protect patients as the healthcare consumers we are. We must switch to a proactive model that protects patients from abuse and fraud through laws that shield us. If we are of value to health insurers only if we're healthy, not if we're accessing their "product," then we need protections when we get sick.

The next step is demanding protections written by patients for patients. We can't wait for industry or politicians to "gift" them. We need a grassroots lobby that fights to lock in protections against predatory practices, not just access to an insurance card. Patients themselves must write the rules, build a lobby, and rig the system in our favor for the first time.

9   We the Patients

Obviously, I love a good pop culture reference to help make sense of a situation, and I can think of no better way to explain where we are in American healthcare's history than to reference *A Bug's Life*, the 1998 Pixar/Disney animated film starring Kevin Spacey as the bad guy, a grasshopper named Hopper.

Every year, Hopper and his gang of grasshoppers shake down a colony of ants for food. Naturally, there's a good guy, an ant and hapless inventor named Flik, played by Dave Foley of *The Kids in the Hall*, who tries to rally the ants to stand up to Hopper. At first, the ants don't see the value in organizing an uprising, and the grasshoppers dismiss the ants as "puny." But Hopper understands what's at stake if they turn on him.

"You let one ant stand up to us, then they might all stand up. Those 'puny little ants' outnumber us a hundred to one, and if they ever figured that out, there goes our way of life!"[1]

It's just so perfect an analogy for the healthcare industry. Maintain power even though they're outnumbered and make money off the "puny" ones who think they have no choice but to comply. But what if we stood up to them like Flik did?

"Ants don't serve grasshoppers. It's you who need us," Flik says to Hopper, whose face reveals his fear of an ant revolution, while all the ants and the grasshoppers look on. "We're a lot stronger than you say we are, and you know it, don't you?"[2] It makes me want to sell rubber wristbands with images of Flik and the words "Stronger and you know it," if I didn't think Disney would slap me with a lawsuit.

We are the ants of American healthcare. It's just hard to feel like we're stronger than we seem, especially after the historic slashing of healthcare through the One Big Beautiful Bill (OBBB) on our nation's birthday in 2025. It nearly broke Rep. Alexandria Ocasio-Cortez (D-NY), who stood on the Capitol steps the day Congress passed the law and said, "I don't think we've ever seen, or are prepared, for how catastrophic this is set to be for a lot of people, and I think it's devastating." She called it the largest blow to healthcare in American history and added that there needed to be real consequences for passing the bill, in the election booth. "I hope people vote like it's our real lives."[3]

While our elected politicians voted to effectively strip millions of Americans of their healthcare and raise costs for millions more, I was thinking about Ralph Nader and seat belts. (See Chapter 8.) The outcome of Nader's consumer protection crusade always struck me as a solid example of consumers and industry both winning at the same time. Industry, because seat belts meant fewer lawsuits and better PR, both which boost the bottom line. Consumers, for dying less. And it made me wonder: Can our for-profit healthcare industry make money without screwing us over?

The social media comedian and ophthalmologist Will Flanary, MD, a.k.a. "Dr. Glaucomflecken," doesn't seem so sure they can. In a tongue-in-cheek video posted in the summer of 2025, he addressed the tired trope that the industry deliberately keeps people sick to make money. In it, Flanary depicts fictional doctors, hospitals, and Big Pharma, but it's health insurance, represented by the comedian holding a UnitedHealthcare binder, that says rather bluntly: "I want people to be completely healthy or dead."[4]

That's because sick people cost Big Insurance money. But if you don't use your health insurance or you just use it for nothing more than your annual check-up and maybe a mysterious rash after that time in a hotel hot tub, you won't even come close to paying down your annual deductible, and your insurance company will pocket your premiums. The moment you reach your deductible, though, you start costing them money, and the meter starts running. Patient protections keep them from pushing you out of the cab.

The way the system runs today, Big Insurance has no incentive to keep you sick because your doctor's visits, tests, procedures, chemo, radiation, and surgeries cut into their bottom line. But they also have no real incentive to make sure you're healthy, either, not when they can delay and deny their way to profits. The system is deliberately packed with friction. This is their business model now.

Except, that's actually pretty expensive. Every year, insurers spend $10.6 billion fighting with patients over unnecessary insurance claim denials, as half of all denied claims are eventually overturned and paid anyhow.[5] Meanwhile, patients sweat it out, as we so often do, with nearly half skipping or delaying care because of the cost.[6]

Yet it's not like we can boycott health insurance. There's no health-care version of Occupy Wall Street or a boycott like cancelling Disney+ to make an expensive point. It doesn't work that way when the product you're fighting over can affect whether or not you live or die or at least ruin your shot at getting healthy.

I began to wonder, what if there were no prior auths, no denials, no medical bankruptcy? Who would make money in this version of a for-profit system? Big Pharma, medical testing facilities, and medical device companies, that's who. Also, hospitals and physicians, though the latter would still be drowning in paperwork. So Big Insurance has gotten into that game, too, buying up hospital systems and medical practices. Now they're double-dipping, making money no matter your health status.

If that sounds horrifically duplicitous, let me remind you that the system isn't broken. It was built this way, and it takes strong guardrails to keep it in check. Let me be clear that I do not believe that any part of the system—least of all, doctors—wants us to stay sick. My own doctors surely wanted to see this college kid survive. But a for-profit healthcare system must make money for it to survive, earnings report by earnings report.

If we take away some of the boondoggles of the system that make them money at our expense, like claim delays and denials, prior auths, and PBM kickbacks, some groups win and some lose, namely insurers and PBMs, but also Medicare Advantage (which *is* Big Insurance) and Medicaid which use prior auths to keep costs down.

Notice that the winners are rarely patients. Winning doesn't just mean not dying or not going broke, though these are our main goals. It also means surviving the system to overcome a disease without sizable out-of-pocket costs, medical debt or bankruptcy, denials, delays, insurance loss, job loss, surprise medical bills, racial disparities and discrimination, billing errors, narrow networks and coverage gaps, and that one medical professional who tells you that you'll never heal until you have an "attitude of gratitude," as though your thoughts are stronger than chemo. (We all know if that were true, Big Insurance would charge us for our thoughts.)

We have always been at the mercy of the system. We don't get to decide what's best for us, just what we can eke out of whatever coverage we have, putting us forever on the defense. If you're lucky, you get to choose a good quality healthcare plan that covers the care you need where you want to get it when you get sick. But if you're employed by someone else, chances are you don't get a choice in that plan, and yet it's still called a "benefit." Meanwhile, only 54 percent of employers even offer health insurance.[7]

If you get your coverage through the ACA, which saw enrollment double between the pandemic and Trump 47,[8] chances are, you are an employee of a company that doesn't offer health insurance, a small business owner, or self-employed.[9] It's also likely that you've received premium tax credits that, thanks to the OBBB, have now gone missing.[10]

Every enrollment period brings surprises, and I don't mean the "Oooh! Cupcakes!" variety. Maybe the price for your plan's premiums went up, or the deductibles cost as much as an Alaskan cruise trip, or the plan no longer exists. Perhaps it's hard to tell the difference between a silver and a bronze plan, and you're not sure the gold is the best option even if it costs a bunch more. You might find that your doctors are suddenly out of network or your [insert expensive medication that keeps your health steady] is no longer covered. Maybe you're on Medicare but you forgot to sign up for Medigap, or you're trapped under a pile of Medicaid paperwork trying to prove you still need and deserve your healthcare.

Meanwhile, somewhere in Canada, someone just left the hospital without a hefty bill.

I'm not even advocating for the pie-in-the-sky idea that America would ever get universal healthcare, though I do fantasize about it. I'm just saying that maybe we shouldn't need a cottage industry of scrappy advocates who help you fight healthcare chicanery for a few grand a pop. And we sure as shit shouldn't need a GoFundMe to pay for chemo.

Imagine if our favorite TV and movie characters had to face the same healthcare malfeasance we do:

- What if on *Friends*, Phoebe's asthma inhaler suddenly quintupled in price from $60 out of pocket to more than $500 because a PBM decided not to cover it anymore?
- What if all the scientists on *The Big Bang Theory* found that the prestigious regional hospital, Cedars-Sinai, was no longer in network on their university health plans?
- What if Kramer got balance-billed for an injury he sustained sliding through Jerry's door on *Seinfeld*? Or if Medicare Advantage rejected Estelle Costanza's knee replacement?
- What if Tony Soprano's sepsis from a gunshot wound wasn't covered because he was shot in New York City and his insurance was only valid across the Hudson River in New Jersey?

- What if *Breaking Bad*'s Walter White, already unable to afford his cancer treatments thanks to his employer's high-deductible plan, suddenly lost his job and therefore his insurance, and then he got a $40,000 air ambulance ride to the hospital after he flipped his RV into a ditch in the desert?

Then these sitcoms and dramas would be more like reality shows.

America treats patients like a nuisance. Cancer survivors, caregivers, and families get buried in denials, bills, and bureaucracy while the system congratulates itself for providing care and then celebrates record-setting quarterly earnings.

Enough is enough.

You Say You Want a Revolution

It's time that patients become the heroes of their own healthcare journeys, the Fliks to the industry's Hopper. Since the late nineties, I've been fighting for patient rights, trying to help people not just survive cancer, but also to survive the system that comes with it. But I can't be at chemo with everyone, and frankly, you wouldn't want me to be because I'd play clips from *Knight Rider* the whole time.

What if instead there were a movement of patients, survivors, and the people who love them to help prevent asininity in the first place? What if there were a way to protect patients, reduce waste in the industry, and save money for everybody?

Now there is: We the Patients. I created it with a whole bunch of badass ants. Our mission is simple. Together, 19 million cancer patients and survivors plus 35 million caregivers would equal the largest healthcare constituency in the country, a unified group of like-minded voters with the same goal: making cancer and the system that develops, delivers, and funds treatments suck less.

The country has never had a single-issue, populist organizing strategy for healthcare rights, allowing us to rally around cost-saving protections that preserve profits while helping cancer patients. With a movement that big, political candidates will have to answer to us. Corporations will have to answer to us. Wall Street will have to answer to us.

Patients vote. Survivors vote. Caregivers vote. And we're tired of being bullied. We're tired of playing defense. We're fed up with lacking the power to make decisions that affect whether or not we live and how we live when we survive. We refuse to accept that our health insurance is what determines whether we live or die, and we are sick and tired of being sick and tired because of the system.

We live by our own Miranda rights:

You have the right to understand your care: every test, every bill, every choice.

You have the right to a human guide who walks beside you, not a call center that leaves you stranded.

You have the right to protection from financial ruin when you are fighting for your life and your health.

You have the right to fight cancer, not bureaucracy.

You have the right to dignity, clarity, and truth in every decision made about your body and your future.

Now more than ever, we need Cancer Advocacy 2.0. It's time to drop your biology, refocus from your favorite fundraiser, and take off your "I had [insert type of cancer]" wristband. This isn't about any one type of cancer, yet there's a single agenda: rigging America's for-profit healthcare system in our favor.

Think about it: There were 174 million registered voters during the 2024 election, and about 65 percent actually voted. Who was Most Likely to Vote? Old white folks, with three-quarters of Caucasians over 65 showing up at the polls.[11] You know who tends to get cancer? People over 65, at about 60 percent.[12] What if they got together with pissed off younger patients and voted like their lives depend on it—because they quite literally do. (See: Chainsaw v. Cancer Research.)

When you think of voting blocs and lobbies that have had an out-sized effect on laws in our country, who do you think of? The NRA, the National Rifle Association. Guess what? There are only about 4 million members in the NRA[13] and yet they've been instrumental in getting pro-gun laws passed and blocking anti-gun legislation throughout their history. They did it by writing the laws they wanted to see passed and finding the politicians who'd move them through the system.

But America doesn't step into the voting booth to pull the lever for healthcare. I didn't vote for PBMs, did you? When the federal government shut down over healthcare in October 2025, could you cast your vote for reinstating Medicaid and extending the ACA subsidies? It's way more complicated than that.

The old school "Hill Days," when patients shared their stories with Congress, aren't enough to influence healthcare law these days, and shame doesn't work anymore on Capitol Hill, not when the Speaker of the House can say with a straight face that the OBBB "strengthens our essential programs like Medicaid for the people who need it the most."[14]

But, what if we had an NRA but for patients' rights, and I don't mean the Luigi kind? A well-funded and powerful lobby that shows up in statehouses and Congress to ensure that legislation protects our rights and therefore, our health.

Unfortunately, you can't fix the system if it's working for the people who own it, and the Hoppers of healthcare do not want to give up their power. Let's not forget that the event program for United-Healthcare's 2024 Investor Conference—the meeting that their CEO was headed to that December morning[i]—touted AI for its "administrative simplification."[15] This, while hospitals were reporting unusually high rates of denials by several big insurers, some who were facing lawsuits over the practice of AI-assisted denials.[16] Though UnitedHealthcare insisted that AI was used only as "a guide" for

---

[i] Murder = bad.

humans to determine the fate of your claim,[17] a ProPublica investigation into the practice found that Cigna doctors denied more than 300,000 requests as "medically unnecessary" over a two-month period, spending an average of 1.2 seconds on each case.[18]

Your health is now worthy of attention for about as long as a lightning strike flash.

"We literally click and submit," a former Cigna doctor told ProPublica. "It takes all of ten seconds to do fifty at a time."[19] Cigna pushed back on the story, while several state insurance regulators took note. The major insurers meanwhile promised Congress they'd "streamline, simplify, and reduce" the prior authorization process,[20] so, I dunno, they'll say "no" faster? How can it be any faster? Oh yeah. Robots.

South Park captured just how laughable the entire healthcare system has become in "Navigating the American Healthcare Industry," when the boys try to get Cartman's weight loss medication covered by his insurance company. A tired-looking claims representative in a dark room filled with piles of paper, typewriters, and clacking dot matrix printers makes a call, hangs up, and tells them it's not covered.

"Who was that?" Kyle asks.

"That was the Medical Director. The Medical Director decides what claims are valid for us to pay for," the claims rep says.

"But you didn't say who the patient was or what was wrong with him," Kyle objects.

"Right. The Medical Director's job is just to say 'no.'"[21]

It's time for the Fifth Healthcare Revolution, the next big shift in healthcare rights. From Mary Lasker shaming President Nixon into endorsing the National Cancer Act in the seventies to 1990s American Disabilities Act protecting us at work to the breast cancer wars and the LIVESTRONG Army to the rise of young adult cancer advocacy in this century, we stand on the shoulders of those who fought for our rights before us. Now it's time for the next generation of patients to take the mantle.

To begin to rig the system in our favor, we ants would need to band together to advocate for laws and regulations that protect patients while still helping the for-profit system make money. President Obama and the Democrats did precisely that when they pushed the ACA through Congress while also giving concessions to health insurers, including abandoning a public, government-run option, raising cost-sharing deductibles and copays (some might argue, taking the "affordable" out of the Affordable Care Act), and scaling back expensive "Cadillac" health plans.

At the same time, patients got several wins—pretty big wins compared to the pre-2010 insurance landscape. But the first Trump administration tried to take all that away by arguing that the ACA is unconstitutionally structured and should be, therefore, rendered invalid altogether.[22] A win for them would have been a tremendous loss for people in the individual insurance market because it would have returned the system to pre-ACA rules when cancer was a "declinable condition"[23] while applying for insurance. In the aftermath of the OBBB, the fate of the ACA is again tenuous and perhaps, so too are the patient protection laws that came with it. Will we all become uninsurable?

Cancer Advocacy 1.0 did a great job of working from inside the system, advancing research funding and policy reforms. They've improved countless lives, and their work matters. Hell, I was part of it.

We the Patients is the next big healthcare hack. It's a different way to think about the whole damn process—as voters, not recipients of care. We need to do what Flik did and flip the script on cancer patients as victims and recognize that the millions who have fought and those still fighting cancer are plenty strong enough to also fight the system that holds their fates in its grasshopper hands. First, we were "victims." Then we became survivors. Now, we are a lobby of concerned healthcare consumers.

We the Patients is a nationwide, nonpartisan, patient-led movement fighting to right the wrongs of healthcare. It's a populist effort designed to educate, advocate, and drive systemic change in the name of patient protections through storytelling, policy engagement, and voter activation. Our mission is to hold policymakers and the healthcare industry accountable and demand that they listen, protect, and respect patients. The numbers tell the story of why America's cancer patients need a movement:

- 98 percent of cancer patients with medical debt had health insurance at the time it was incurred[24]
- 96 percent of oncologists say prior authorization has led to delays in cancer treatment[25]
- One-third of cancer patients face insurance denials during active treatment[26]
- One-third of oncologists say prior authorizations have led to patient deaths[27]
- 50 percent of cancer patients have medical debt, and for half of those, the amount exceeds $5,000[28]
- 2 in 5 cancer patients deplete their life savings within two years of diagnosis[29]
- More than one-third of crowdfunding campaigns are for medical reasons[30]

It's time we shift the power in healthcare. We do not ask for awareness. I mean, does anyone really NOT KNOW that cancer exists? We demand accountability. Our nonpartisan campaign organizes patients, caregivers, and allies into a civic force. Together, we will turn lived experience into leverage that lawmakers and industry cannot ignore.

Millions of us—cancer patients and beyond—are exhausted, angry, and pushed to the edge by a system that gaslights, bankrupts, and abandons us while calling it care. We the Patients is a collective scream from a country in pain.

We stand on the shoulders of other patient rights movements:

ACT UP made silence equal death, using civil disobedience and protests to demand research funding, quicker drug approvals, and an end to the stigma of AIDS.

The Breast Cancer Wars turned rage into research, shifting from a medical practice typically limited to radical mastectomy for all to the ubiquitous pinkification of research funding,[31] fundraising, and October.

LIVESTRONG took survivorship mainstream, putting trendy yellow wristbands on celebrities and athletes, humanizing cancer survivors while supporting them.

Stupid Cancer organized millions, giving a generation of patients its voice while reminding us that cancer isn't just geriatric or pediatric.

At We the Patients, our mission is simple: enforce patient rights, hold power to account, and build a system that serves the people living through it.

"We don't need another feel-good, 'Let's develop materials so that you understand your disease,' nonprofit," said We the Patients co-founder Matt Toresco, a healthcare leader, author, speaker, and founder and CEO of Archo Advocacy, LLC. We two Matts are sort of clouds and dirt, my kite to his anchor, the creative and business together in one unit. We may come at it from different angles, but we have the same goal.

"We need patients to know how screwed up the system is," Matt said, "and to be willing to say, "You know what? I don't want that anymore. I want to change it.""

"We need patient representation," he added. "We need people that are willing to be in the trenches alongside patients." Matt has endured his own healthcare fuckery in the form of eleven major spinal surgeries and nearly two decades of being blocked from the surgery that finally relieved him of his chronic pain, all the while being prescribed opioids. He is on board with starting our movement in the cancer community because, "If it's not good for one patient group, it's not good for all of them."

No matter your diagnosis, on day one, you are suddenly hurled into this system that doesn't make sense, and you have to figure it out on the fly. But that's often how patients get overwhelmed and taken advantage of emotionally and financially.

"Healthcare is economics," Matt explained, adding that America has let the healthcare monopoly grow. "Why don't we consider going to the doctor a financial transaction?"

We the Patients focuses on consumer protections first and foremost, and education is protection. It reminds me of the old Syms men's clothing store commercials from the eighties, where Brooklyn-born "Sy Syms" (née Seymour Merinsky) assured those of us watching him during televised New York Giants games, that "An educated consumer is our best customer."[32]

Likewise, an educated patient is the best candidate to protect patient rights and change the system. Not just change it but keep a close eye on the Whack-a-mole game the industry plays in which one anti-patient problem gets knocked down and another pops up, usually in the form of some clever but diabolical workaround that lines the industry's pockets.

Patients are done waiting for scraps of a system that is increasingly working against their favor. We the Patients turns outrage into action, stories into policy, and voters into a bloc powerful enough to change the healthcare system. We invite every cancer patient and the people who love them to join us. The real Revolution happens when patients are in charge of their own outcomes. Together, we are stronger and you know it.

10 We the Revolution

Thirty years after cancer, I still fear the healthcare shitshow because you never know what you're going to get. The late effects of excising a tumor from my brain and radiating my head and neck continue to pop up, throwing me back into the system for tests and procedures. I never know if it'll go smoothly or if I'll be shouting "Representative!" at my health insurance company's automated phone service.

I was fortunate enough to marry into good-ish insurance. My wife, Jessica, gets our health insurance through her job as a school-based speech pathologist, and it covers the hospital where I get my follow-up care. Her plan had been pretty much the same, with the same offerings and guidelines, since 2011. Then, in the summer of 2023, somebody changed the plan, screwing over 3,000 employees and their families in the process.

I'd been taking a medication for terrible reflux, a late effect of the Fukushima-level radiation that left my duodenum, the part of the small intestine that connects to the stomach, in shambles. I'd tried many meds—first Rolaids, then Tums, then Pepcid, then Prilosec, then Nexium—but none of them worked until I found Dexilant, a proton pump inhibitor. It was on my pharmacy's formulary, and my insurance covered it even after the less costly and, for me, less effective generic came out.

My oncology team kept renewing my prescription, and eventually, I started getting my meds mailed to me in an Amazon PillPack. Everything was going great until the day after our insurance changed.

Jessica's employer's insurance plan refused to cover the Dexilant brand-name medication. They refused to cover the generic, though that one didn't work well for me anyhow. They forced me to go through step therapy, where I'd have to try and fail all the meds I'd long ago tried and failed, while my stomach churned and acid built up. I felt sick again. As my friend Sally Neely Nix said about disease, "It does not pause while authorizations are reconsidered or reclassified."

My primary care doctor went to bat for me, filling out the forms for prior authorizations and appeals, but nothing would persuade the pharmacy benefits manager, CVS Caremark, in charge of our plan's formulary. They declared Dexilant medically unnecessary and denied the prescription.

So, I started buying it direct from Canada for $350 for a 90-day supply. Now I was paying $1,400 a year out of pocket for the one medication I've known to work. Lucky for me, my four other meds, including a brain seizure drug, were covered. But when it came to Dexilant, they wouldn't budge.

Then one day, a pharmacist friend mentioned the Pharmacists Society of the State of New York. I sent an email to their executive director, cc-ing my friend, asking for help as a citizen of New York State. I explained the runaround that CVS Caremark had given me, the prior auth denials, the failed appeals, and the unsuccessful third-party appeal. I even shared my LinkedIn plea for advice from my industry insider friends, who provided solid advice involving stuff like override codes and insurance company case managers.

But then my primary care doctor called: she'd gotten the brand approved. The copay would be $150 for a 90-day prescription, saving me $200 a pop. Better, but not really "covered," right?

After all that, my wife's company changed insurance plans again. Now my copay is down to $110 for 90 days but at least I don't have to battle PBMs anymore. It's such a common example of the unnecessary nonsense, and medical and financial harm, that we Americans endure because of our healthcare system.

Yet every once in a while, it all goes right.

Some twenty-eight years after brain surgery, I started getting double vision. I'd never experienced it before. Then Jessica noticed that my left pupil was permanently dilated.

Oh, shit. I thought. *I've got a brain tumor again.* Never mind that there's no chance of a recurrence of a brain tumor you're born with. A "born again" medulloblastoma is not a thing. But once you've had cancer, you assume that every startling new symptom is another cancer.

It happened the year my wife's insurance changed, so my usual hospital where I'd gotten care since the Clinton administration, wasn't covered. Of course. I went to a different hospital where I happened to know the head of the cancer survivorship program,[i] and she hooked me up with an oncologist who ordered an MRI.

I got the doctor's appointment and the MRI without any friction from our insurance company. That was almost as lucky as the outcome: no tumor.

Then we wondered if I'd had another stroke. So, my doctor ordered a CT scan.

Again, my insurance company didn't get in the way.

No evidence of stroke.

Okay, what about an aneurysm? They can cause weird eye problems. It's possible.

So, I had an MRA, a magnetic resonance angiogram, which is a type of MRI that checks the blood vessels.

No delays or denials from my insurance, and the test was clear.

All of these tests were covered, but we still didn't have an answer for what ailed me. The doctor batted around a diagnosis of some sort of electrical glitch caused by radiation that had led to adult

---

[i] Yes, I am aware this is a perk of being me.

strabismus, when one eye is turned in a different direction from the other. It's most commonly found in children, and it's pretty rare in adults. Both my eyes were facing the same direction, but we were running out of ideas.

So, I had to find the nichest of niche specialists: a strabismus surgeon who operates on adults. First, I went to an ophthalmologist, who referred me to a neuro-ophthalmologist, who sent me to a pediatric neuro-ophthalmic surgeon. Fun fact: she was located just a block from Stupid Cancer's headquarters. She did a bunch of tests and then she told me to wait four months to see if it gets worse because if it did, that would warrant a particular type of surgery.

All of those specialists and all of those tests were covered.

My eye didn't get worse. It just got really annoying, interfering with my everyday life. When I played the piano, I couldn't see my right hand as it traveled up the keys. I had to stop driving, and I would tell my kids I could see two of each of them, but I wasn't sure which one was talking. And because they're my kids, they would play along. "I'm over here, Dad."

On the day of the surgery, I had to pay $7,000 up front to cover our annual deductible, and I put it on a credit card. But now we were back on the original insurance plan, which has a health reimbursement arrangement that would pay us back later. We got it all back, minus $750 for the surgery copay.

I had the surgery and now I am completely cured. But I never once had to shout at my insurance company. No one along the way ever uttered the words "medically unnecessary." No one blocked me from care or tests. Nobody made me try other therapies first. Nobody called the surgery "elective" or "cosmetic," and no one sent me an outrageous and unexpected bill.

In all, I paid about $1,000 in copays and deductibles, in addition to our premiums, and—here's the important part—my eye works just fine. My kids no longer appear to have doubled, I can drive again, and I can even see my right hand when I play the piano.

This is what it's like when the American healthcare system works. It's my testimony to how it can make money for the system while also helping patients. Imagine if navigating our healthcare system was always this seamless, if patients got healthy while the system made money and nobody needed to find another workaround. Then the healthcare fuckery would finally be over.

But for that to happen in today's America, it's going to take a revolution of patients who have had enough.

About the Authors

Matthew Zachary has spent three decades fighting to make the American healthcare system less cruel, organizing millions through advocacy and media. A former concert pianist whose life was turned upside down by brain cancer at just 21, he founded Stupid Cancer, the largest nonprofit for young adults with cancer. He also launched The Stupid Cancer Show, widely regarded as the first healthcare podcast, which later evolved into the award-winning Out of Patients. He produced Cancer Mavericks, a documentary series about the rebel patients who changed modern oncology. He is CEO and Co-Founder of We The Patients, a national movement organizing patients into collective civic power.

Jen Singer is a bestselling ghostwriter and editor, and the author of *The Just Diagnosed Guides*. She has survived cancer, a complete heart block, and the American healthcare system.

Acknowledgments

Thank you to the universe for letting me live. I have no idea why I made it. Maybe there is a reason. Maybe not. Either way, I am still here.

To my wife, Jessica Feldman. You have stood by every version of me without fail. To my miracle children, Koby and Hannah. You are my reason for breathing.

To my parents. You created me, raised me, tolerated me, and kept doing it. To my brother, my sister-in-law, my nieces, and my nephew. The connection may stretch, but it never breaks.

To my in-laws, Hinda and Jerry Feldman. You have become the family I never knew I needed. To my late brother-in-law Karl Feldman. You were taken before your time but inspired so many lives. To my Aunt Natalie and Uncle Marty. You are proof that blood is thicker than geography. To my cousin Emily Stein, Robbie Stein, and their family. Thank you for your endless love and support. To my late cousin, Rabbi David Stein, who married my wife and me and faced brain cancer with grace.

To my Uncle Jay Tischfield. You made sure my medical choices were mine and no one else's.

To the people who gave me a future: Dr. Ehud Arbit, my neurosurgeon, Dr. Jeffrey Allen and the NYU Hassenfeld team, Dr. Thomas Merchant and Dr. Brian Davis from Sloan Kettering, now at St Jude and the Mayo Clinic. Every nurse, resident, and orderly who kept me alive the week of January 9, 1996. Every friend who walked through that hospital room door. I remember. So many "Get Well" balloons.

To my gaggle of old-school legacy 1980s BFFs: Phil Eisenberg, John DeMarco, Laura Larkin, Suzanne McFeeley. To my 1990s college BFFs: Brian Friedman, Adam Price, Jason Price, Mara Hitner, and to my oldest standing friend from first grade, Dr. Jennifer Stein. And to anyone who visited me in the hospital in 1996 during that uncertain week amidst a blizzard. You helped keep me alive.

To summer camp. Lots of mixed feelings, but you taught me more about resilience, survival, and self-worth than any classroom ever could. It made me who I am. To every teacher from kindergarten through college. You taught lessons that went far beyond the subject. To Mrs. Bertha Mandel, my first piano teacher, who taught me discipline, structure, and the framework for musicianship.

To Binghamton University. You bent every rule so I could graduate when life exploded. To Sarah Armstrong, my "old friend" and my musical theater soulmate, who made sure I kept pointing in the right direction for myself, in love and in life. To the late Professor Susan J. Peters, who saw potential when I could not and opened my world with a stern grip to infinite creative possibilities.

To Craig Lustig, my first "cancer buddy" who showed me the way, who turned the chaos of experience into a map for advocacy. To the late Ellen Stovall and the late Selma Schimmel. You were the architects of my purpose. Ellen, you were a luminary in survivorship and cancer advocacy. You taught me how to turn survival into mission and mission into movement. Selma, you helped give birth to my broadcast career and made me the "podfather" of healthcare before the word podcast even existed. To the framers of the LIVESTRONG Young Adult Alliance, who gave a generation its foundation.

To Dr. Leonard Sender, my first Board Chair who showed me there can be true leadership in young adult cancer advocacy. To Kenny Kane, my co-founder of Stupid Cancer. My rock. My brother. My best friend. My family. Our secrets will die with us. You are an anchor in this space and in my life. To Elizabeth Woolfe, my Jiminy Cricket, Sherpa, big sister therapist, conscience of Stupid Cancer, and work best friend. You kept me honest, grounded, and human.

To every volunteer, sponsor, and mentor who helped build Stupid Cancer. To the early donors and believers who turned an idea into a movement.

To every nonprofit partner, corporate ally, and every work wife, work husband, and work spouse who kept showing up.

To Jen Singer, who helped me put this story on paper.

To Christina Verigan, who made sure the words looked great. To my publisher, Wiley, who believed it mattered. To Scott Kaufman at Buchwald, who fought for it. To Ben Press, who set it all in motion. To Lia Aponte, who kept me sane and grounded.

To everyone who contributed to this book. Every voice. Every story. Every insight. To Wendell Potter for your integrity and honesty. To Christy Snodgrass, Monica Bryant, Candice Roth, and Shelley Fuld Nasso for your candor, brilliance, and moral conviction. You gave this book its backbone. Thank you for trusting me with your truth.

To Sally Neely Nix, Matt Toresco, and Maimah Karmo. You helped form We The Patients with me and turned a spark into a movement. You believed in the idea before it had a name.

To the entire cancer community: Patients. Caregivers. Nonprofit leaders. Clinicians. Advocates. You prove every day that survival is a team sport. To everyone who ever listened, read, shared, or cared. You kept the lights on. And finally, to Mark Cuban who makes my job easier every time he opens his mouth.

To everyone who ignored me, bullied me, ghosted me, doubted me, or said no. You made the yeses matter.

To whatever force keeps me upright, loud, and useful. Thank you. You made it to the credits.

Notes

Preface

1. David U. Himmelstein, Robert M. Lawless, Deborah Thorne, Pamela Foohey, and Steffie Woolhandler, "Medical Bankruptcy: Still Common Despite the Affordable Care Act," *American Journal of Public Health* 109, no. 3 (March 2019): 431–433, accessed October 6, 2025, https://pmc.ncbi.nlm.nih.gov/articles/PMC6366487/. (PubMed).
2. David Crosby et al., "Early Detection of Cancer," *Science* 375, no. 6586 (March 18, 2022): eaay9040, https://doi.org/10.1126/science.aay9040.
3. Emily Tonorezos et al., "Prevalence of Cancer Survivors in the United States," *Journal of the National Cancer Institute* 116, no. 11 (2024): 1784–1790, https://doi.org/10.1093/jnci/djae135. (pubmed.ncbi.nlm.nih.gov).

Chapter 1

1. Social Security Administration, Health Maintenance Organization Act of 1973, Notes and Brief Reports, *Social Security Bulletin* 37, no. 3 (March 1974): 35–39, https://www.ssa.gov/policy/docs/ssb/v37n3/v37n3p35.pdf.
2. Robert James Cimasi, *Healthcare Valuation: The Four Pillars of Healthcare Value, Volume 1* (Hoboken, NJ: John Wiley & Sons, 2014), 50.
3. John Kruzel, "No, It Was Not Illegal to Profit off U.S. Healthcare before a Nixon-Era Law," PolitiFact, May 1, 2019, https://www.politifact.com/factchecks/2019/may/01/blog-posting/no-it-was-not-illegal-profit-us-healthcare-nixon-e/.
4. U.S. Government Accountability Office, *Financial Audit: FY 2021 and FY 2020 Consolidated Financial Statements of the U.S. Government, GAO-22-105122* (Washington, D.C.: U.S. Government Accountability Office, February 17, 2022), https://www.gao.gov/products/gao-22-105122.

5. American Association of Colleges of Nursing, *Nursing Shortage Fact Sheet* (Washington, DC: AACN, May 2024), https://www.aacnnursing.org/Portals/0/PDFs/Fact-Sheets/Nursing-Shortage-Factsheet.pdf.

6. Flip Timotija, "Mangione Defense Fund Tops $1M," *The Hill*, May 6, 2025, https://www.thehill.com/regulation/court-battles/5285980-luigi-mangione-fundraiser/.

7. UnitedHealth Group, *UnitedHealth Group Reports 2024 Results*, January 16, 2025, https://www.unitedhealthgroup.com/content/dam/UHG/PDF/investors/2024/2025-16-01-uhg-reports-fourth-quarter-results.pdf.

8. Erica Kollmann, "UnitedHealth Investors Claim Company Hid Profit Impact of CEO's Murder," *Benzinga*, May 8, 2025, https://www.benzinga.com/general/health-care/25/05/45305392/unitedhealth-investors-claim-company-hid-profit-impact-of-ceos-murder.

9. Kollmann, "UnitedHealth Investors Claim Company Hid Profit Impact of CEO's Murder."

10. Senate Permanent Subcommittee on Investigations, U.S. Senate, "Senate Permanent Subcommittee on Investigations Releases Majority Staff Report Exposing Medicare Advantage Insurers' Refusal of Care for Vulnerable Seniors," press release, October 17, 2024, Blumenthal.senate.gov, https://www.blumenthal.senate.gov/newsroom/press/release/senate-permanent-subcommittee-on-investigations-releases-majority-staff-report-exposing-medicare-advantage-insurers-refusal-of-care-for-vulnerable-seniors.

11. David U. Himmelstein et al., "Medical Bankruptcy: Still Common Despite the Affordable Care Act," *American Journal of Public Health* 109, no. 3 (February 6, 2019): e1–e5, https://doi.org/10.2105/ajph.2018.304901.

12. Joseph S. Ross, "The Committee on the Costs of Medical Care and the History of Health Insurance in the United States," *Einstein Quarterly Journal of Biology and Medicine* 19 (2002): 129–134.

13. Physicians for a National Health Program, "A Brief History: Universal Health Care Efforts in the US," *PNHP*, accessed September 23, 2025, https://pnhp.org/a-brief-history-universal-health-care-efforts-in-the-us/.

14. Joseph S. Ross, "The Committee on the Costs of Medical Care and the History of Health Insurance in the United States," *Einstein Quarterly Journal of Biology and Medicine* 19 (2002): 129–134, https://einsteinmed.edu/uploadedFiles/EJBM/19Ross129.pdf.

15. Ross, "The Committee on the Costs of Medical Care and the History of Health Insurance in the United States," 130.

16. Thomas B. Gore, "A Forgotten Landmark Medical Study from 1932 by the Committee on the Cost of Medical Care," *Proceedings (Baylor University*

Medical Center) 26, no. 2 (2013): 142–143, https://pmc.ncbi.nlm.nih.gov/articles/PMC3603728.

17. "Socialized Medicine Is Urged in Survey," *The New York Times*, November 30, 1932, TimesMachine, https://timesmachine.nytimes.com/timesmachine/1932/11/30/105889886.html?pageNumber=1.

18. Ross, *"The Committee on the Costs of Medical Care and the History of Health Insurance in the United States,"* 132.

19. "The Committee on the Costs of Medical Care Presents Its Final Report," *Milbank Memorial Quarterly* 11, no. 1 (1933): 1-10, https://www.milbank.org/wp-content/uploads/mq/volume-11/issue-01/11-1-The-Committee-on-the-Costs-of-Medical-Care-Presents-in-Final-Report.pdf.

20. "The Committee on the Costs of Medical Care," *JAMA* 99, no. 23 (1932): 1950-1952, 10.1001/jama.1932.02740750052015.

21. "Committee on the Costs of Medical Care Presents Its Final Report," *Milbank Memorial Quarterly* 11, no. 1 (1933).

22. David Blumenthal, "Employer-Sponsored Health Insurance in the United States — Origins and Implications," *The New England Journal of Medicine* 355, no. 1 (July 6, 2006): 82, https://people.umass.edu/econ340/nejm-ebhi.pdf.

23. Blumenthal, "Employer-Sponsored Health Insurance," 82.

24. U.S. Senate, *Congressional Record*, 79th Cong., 1st sess., vol. 91, pt. 8 (November 19, 1945): 10794, https://www.govinfo.gov/content/pkg/GPO-CRECB-1945-pt8/pdf/GPO-CRECB-1945-pt8-22-1.pdf.

25. PNHP, "A Brief History: Universal Health Care Efforts in the US."

26. Ibid.

27. Sheila Mulrooney Eldred, "When Harry Truman Pushed for Universal Health Care," *History*, November 12, 2019, A&E Television Networks, https://www.history.com/articles/harry-truman-universal-health-care.

28. Dan Gorenstein, "How Did We End Health Insurance Being Tied to Our Jobs?" *Marketplace.org*, June 28, 2017, https://www.marketplace.org/story/2017/06/28/how-did-we-end-health-insurance-being-tied-our-jobs.

29. U.S. Bureau of the Census, *Census of Population, 1970, Part 1: Series B 401-412, Chapter B: Vital Statistics, Including Statistics of Births, Deaths, Marriages, and Divorces, Series B 1-220* (Washington, D.C.: U.S. Government Printing Office, 1970), https://www2.census.gov/prod2/statcomp/documents/CT1970p1-03.pdf.

30. Melissa A. Thomasson, "Racial Differences in Health Insurance Coverage and Medical Expenditures in the United States: A Historical Perspective," *The Milbank Quarterly* 78, no. 3 (2000): 385-415, https://www.jstor.org/stable/40267921.

31. David Blumenthal, "Employer-Sponsored Health Insurance in the United States—Origins and Implications," *New England Journal of Medicine* 355, no. 1 (July 6, 2006): 88, https://doi.org/10.1056/NEJMhpr060703.

32. Tom van der Voort, "In the Beginning: Medicare and Medicaid," *Miller Center*, August 4, 2017, https://millercenter.org/issues-policy/us-domestic-policy/beginning-medicare-and-medicaid.

33. van der Voort, "In the Beginning: Medicare and Medicaid."

34. Kate Stalter, "Why Older Citizens Are More Likely to Vote," *U.S. News & World Report*, n.d., https://money.usnews.com/money/retirement/aging/articles/why-older-citizens-are-more-likely-to-vote.

35. "A Brief History of Medicare in America," *MedicareResources.org*, accessed September 23, 2025, https://www.medicareresources.org/basic-medicare-information/brief-history-of-medicare.

36. "Harry and Louise on Clinton's Health Plan," YouTube video, 3:27, posted by [danieljbmitchell], [July 15, 2007], https://www.youtube.com/watch?v=Dt31nhleeCg.

37. Chris Riotta, "GOP Aims To Kill Obamacare Yet Again After Failing 70 Times," *Newsweek*, July 29, 2017, https://www.newsweek.com/gop-health-care-bill-repeal-and-replace-70-failed-attempts-643832.

38. Victoria Knight, "Back to the Future: Trump's History of Promising a Health Plan That Never Comes," *KFF Health News*, August 13, 2020, https://kffhealthnews.org/news/back-to-the-future-trumps-history-of-promising-a-health-plan-that-never-comes/.

39. "Trump's Medicaid Cuts Revealed: 'Big Beautiful Bill' Could Leave Millions Without Medical Care," *FastCompany*, May 12, 2025, https://www.fastcompany.com/91332570/trumps-medicaid-cuts-revealed-big-beautiful-bill-leave-millions-without-medical-care.

40. Statista, "Total Medicaid Expenditure Since 1966," Statista.com, accessed September 23, 2025, https://www.statista.com/statistics/245348/total-medicaid-expenditure-since-1966.

41. William H. Dow, "What Do the Looming Cuts to Medicaid Really Mean?," *UC Berkeley School of Public Health Commentary*, July 22, 2025, https://publiche alth.berkeley.edu/articles/news/commentary/what-do-cuts-to-medicaid-really-mean/?utm_source=chatgpt.com.

42. Rebecca Robbins and Reed Abelson, "Why Patients Are Being Forced to Switch to a 2nd-Choice Obesity Drug," *The New York Times*, May 11, 2025, https://www.nytimes.com/2025/05/11/health/zepbound-wegovy-weight-loss-drugs.html.

43. Louis J. Aronne et al., "Tirzepatide as Compared with Semaglutide for the Treatment of Obesity," *New England Journal of Medicine* 393, no. 1 (July 3, 2025): 26-36, https://doi.org/10.1056/NEJMoa2416394.
44. Robbins and Abelson, "Why Patients Are Being Forced to Switch to a 2nd-Choice Obesity Drug," *New York Times*.
45. Ibid.
46. Wendell Potter and Joey Rettino, "Big Shifts: CVS Is Pulling the Plug on ACA Coverage—And 1 Million Americans Will Pay the Price," *HEALTH CARE Uncovered(Substack)*, May 15, 2025.

Chapter 2

1. American Medical Association, "Trends in Health Care Spending," AMA, accessed September 27, 2025, https://www.ama-assn.org/about/ama-research/trends-health-care-spending?utm_source=chatgpt.com.
2. Kaiser Family Foundation, "National Health Expenditures Per Capita, 1960–2023," *KFF*, accessed September 27, 2025, https://www.kff.org/health-costs/slide/national-health-expenditures-per-capita-1960-2023/?utm_source=chatgpt.com.
3. "Titans Vs Mighty Insurance Snake," *Teen Titans Go!*, video, 1:30, uploaded by *Cartoon Network*, April 5, 2022, YouTube video, https://www.youtube.com/watch?v=jTijLfSwsNQ.
4. University of Rochester Medical Center, "Trigeminal Neuralgia," URMC, accessed September 27, 2025, https://www.urmc.rochester.edu/conditions-and-treatments/trigeminal-neuralgia.
5. Lauren Sausser, "Doctors and Patients Try to Shame Insurers Online to Reverse Prior Authorization Denials," *KFF Health News*, accessed September 27, 2025, https://kffhealthnews.org/news/article/doctors-patients-shame-insurers-online-prior-authorization-denials/?utm_source=chatgpt.com.
6. "Don't Let Profit Deny Patients Their Right to Healthcare – Petition HCSC NOW!," *Change.org*, accessed September 27, 2025, https://www.change.org/p/don-t-let-profit-deny-patients-their-right-to-healthcare-petition-hcsc-now?utm_source=chatgpt.com.
7. U.S. Department of Labor, "Employee Retirement Income Security Act (ERISA)," accessed September 27, 2025, https://www.dol.gov/general/topic/retirement/erisa.
8. Sally Nix, LinkedIn post (Nov. 2023), accessed September 27, 2025, https://www.linkedin.com/posts/sallynix_healthcare-facts-bluecrossblueshieldillinois-activity-7112486135284584448-bj6e?utm_source=share&utm_medium=member_desktop&rcm=ACoAAAAtCskBVrYQ_HMUtGpmYB_69xMXaEGpX2Q.

9. Worldometer, "Life Expectancy," accessed September 27, 2025, https://www.worldometers.info/demographics/life-expectancy/.

10. American Medical Association, "What Is Prior Authorization?" *AMA*, accessed September 27, 2025, https://www.ama-assn.org/practice-management/prior-authorization/what-prior-authorization.

11. Jacqueline LaPointe, "Prior Authorizations Often Denied, Adding to Provider Burden," *TechTarget*, June 24, 2024, https://www.techtarget.com/revcycle management/news/366600103/Prior-authorizations-often-denied-adding-to-provider-burden.

12. Patrick Rucker, Maya Miller, and David Armstrong, "How Cigna Saves Millions by Having Its Doctors Reject Claims Without Reading Them," ProPublica, March 25, 2023, https://www.propublica.org/article/cigna-pxdx-medical-health-insurance-rejection-claims.

13. American Medical Association, *Prior Authorization Survey* (Chicago, IL: AMA, n.d.), accessed September 27, 2025, https://www.ama-assn.org/system/files/prior-authorization-survey.pdf.

14. "Utilization Review & Medical Necessity," *McG Health* Blog, June 21, 2018, accessed September 27, 2025, https://www.mcg.com/blog/2018/06/21/utilization-review-medical-necessity/.

15. "Utilization Review & Medical Necessity."

16. American Medical Association, *Prior Authorization Survey*.

17. Healthinsurance.org, "Prior Authorization," accessed September 27, 2025, https://www.healthinsurance.org/glossary/prior-authorization/.

18. Robin Fields, "How Often Do Health Insurers Deny Patients' Claims? No One Knows," ProPublica, June 28, 2023, accessed September 27, 2025, https://www.propublica.org/article/how-often-do-health-insurers-deny-patients-claims.

19. "Health Insurance Denial Rates by Company," *Wallace Insurance Law Blog*, April 18, 2025, accessed September 27, 2025, https://www.wallaceinsurancelaw.com/health-insurance-denial-rates-by-company/?utm.

20. Karen Pollitz, Justin Lo, Rayna Wallace, and Salem Mengistu, "Claims Denials and Appeals in ACA Marketplace Plans in 2021," *KFF* (issue brief, February 9, 2023), accessed September 27, 2025, https://www.kff.org/private-insurance/issue-brief/claims-denials-and-appeals-in-aca-marketplace-plans/.

21. Ibid.

22. @drelisabethpotter, Instagram post January 7, 2025, accessed September 27, 2025, https://www.instagram.com/p/DEid-1npNbA/?hl=en.

23. Kara Nesvig, "A Plastic Surgeon's Clash With an Insurance Company Touches a Nerve," *Allure*, February 27, 2025, accessed September 27, 2025, https://www.allure.com/story/elisabeth-potter-united-healthcare.

24. Bevan Hurley, "Dr Elisabeth Potter: I Criticised UnitedHealth – Now I'm Facing Ruin," *The Times*, July 16, 2025, accessed September 27, 2025, https://www.thetimes.com/us/news-today/article/elisabeth-potter-united-health-dr-bill-ackman-surgeon-x330l6wxc?region=global.

25. *Class Action v. UnitedHealth and NaviHealth*, PDF, accessed September 27, 2025, https://cdn.arstechnica.net/wp-content/uploads/2023/11/class-action-v-unitedhealth-and-navihealth-1.pdf.

26. Grace Sparks, Julian Montalvo III, Shannon Schumacher, Ashley Kirzinger, and Liz Hamel, "KFF Health Tracking Poll: Public Finds Prior Authorization Process Difficult to Manage," *KFF*, July 25, 2025, accessed September 27, 2025, https://www.kff.org/patient-consumer-protections/poll-finding/kff-health-tracking-poll-public-finds-prior-authorization-process-difficult-to-manage/.

27. Justin Lo, Michelle Long, Rayna Wallace, Meghan Salaga, and Kaye Pestaina, "Claims Denials and Appeals in ACA Marketplace Plans in 2023," *KFF*, January 27, 2025, accessed September 27, 2025, https://www.kff.org/private-insurance/claims-denials-and-appeals-in-aca-marketplace-plans-in-2023/. (kff.org).

28. Sarah Kliff, "Health Insurers Are Denying More Drug Claims, Data Shows," *The New York Times*, July 18, 2025, accessed September 27, 2025, https://www.nytimes.com/2025/07/18/health/health-insurance-prescription-claim-denials.html.

29. "The 1960s," in *The Pharmaceutical Century*, accessed September 27, 2025, https://farmamol.web.uah.es/The%20Pharmaceutical%20Century/Ch5.html.

30. "The 1960s," in *The Pharmaceutical Century*.

31. Thomas R. Oliver, Philip R. Lee, and Helene L. Lipton, "A Political History of Medicare and Prescription Drug Coverage," *Milbank Quarterly* 82, no. 2 (June 2004): 283–354, https://pmc.ncbi.nlm.nih.gov/articles/PMC2690175/.

32. "PBM Basics," *Pharmaceutical Society of the State of New York*, accessed September 27, 2025, https://www.pssny.org/page/PBMBasics.

33. "PBM Basics."

34. "Final Investigative Report: Pharmacy Benefit Managers in New York," New York State Senate Committee on Investigations and Government Operations and Committee on Health, May 31, 2019, accessed September 27, 2025, https://www.nysenate.gov/sites/default/files/article/attachment/final_investigatory_report_pharmacy_benefit_managers_in_new_york.pdf. (nysenate.gov).

35. "PBM Basics."

36. Ibid.

37. "Final Investigative Report: Pharmacy Benefit Managers in New York."

38. "The Need for Legislation Regarding "Maximum Allowable Cost" (MAC) Reimbursement," National Community Pharmacists Association, accessed September 27, 2025, https://www.ncpa.co/pdf/leg/mac-one-pager.pdf.

39. Frier Levitt, LLC, *White Paper on PBM DIR Fees: Investigative White Paper on Background, Cost Impact, and Legal Issues* (commissioned by Community Oncology Alliance, January 2017), accessed September 27, 2025, https://communityoncology.org/wp-content/uploads/2017/01/COA_White_Paper_on_DIR-Final.pdf.

40. Jessica Wapner, "Understanding the Hidden Villain of Big Pharma: Pharmacy Benefit Managers," *Newsweek*, March 17, 2017, updated July 27, 2017, accessed September 27, 2025, https://www.newsweek.com/big-pharma-villain-pbm-569980.

41. "The Three Ways PBMs Make Money: Rebates, Admin Fees and Spread," AffirmedRx, accessed September 27, 2025, https://affirmedrx.com/how-pbms-make-money/.

42. Zach Freed, "The Pharmacy Benefit Mafia: The Secret Health Care Monopolies Jacking Up Drug Prices and Abusing Patients and Pharmacists," *American Economic Liberties Project*, June 22, 2022, accessed September 27, 2025, https://www.economicliberties.us/our-work/the-pharmacy-benefit-mafia-the-secret-health-care-monopolies-jacking-up-drug-prices-and-abusing-patients-and-pharmacists/.

43. Stacy Mitchell and Zach Freed, "How the FTC Protected the Market Power of Pharmacy Benefit Managers," *ProMarket*, February 19, 2021, accessed September 27, 2025, https://www.promarket.org/2021/02/19/ftc-market-power-pharmacy-benefit-managers/.

44. "FTC Sues Prescription Drug Middlemen for Artificially Inflating Insulin Drug Prices," Federal Trade Commission, September 20, 2024, accessed September 27, 2025, https://www.ftc.gov/news-events/news/press-releases/2024/09/ftc-sues-prescription-drug-middlemen-artificially-inflating-insulin-drug-prices.

45. Erik P. Eckholm, Solving America's Health-Care Crisis: A Guide to Understanding the Greatest Threat to Your Family's Economic Security (New York: Times Books, 1993), accessed via Internet Archive, page 302, https://archive.org/details/solvingamericash00eckh/page/302/mode/2up.

46. Eckholm, Solving America's Health-Care Crisis, 304.

47. "Pres. Clinton's Address to Congress on Health Care (1993)," YouTube video, 1:12:45, posted by *clintonlibrary42*, September 22, 2011, accessed September 27, 2025, https://www.youtube.com/watch?v=3K1d3E-BoUw&t=1282s.

48. "Pres. Clinton's Address to Congress on Health Care (1993)."

49. Adam Clymer, "The Nation: The Clinton Health Plan Is Alive on Arrival," *New York Times*, October 3, 1993, accessed September 27, 2025, https://www.nytimes.com/1993/10/03/weekinreview/the-nation-the-clinton-health-plan-is-alive-on-arrival.html.

50. "Contract with America," *U-S-History.com*, accessed September 27, 2025, https://www.u-s-history.com/pages/h2052.html.

51. Theda Skocpol, *"The Time Is Never Ripe: The Repeated Defeat of Universal Health Insurance in the Twentieth Century United States"* (Geary Lecture 26, 1995; Dublin: The Economic and Social Research Institute), accessed September 27, 2025, https://www.esri.ie/system/files/publications/GLS26.pdf.

52. Ronald Brownstein, "THE TIMES POLL: By 2–1 Margin, Public Backs Health Care Plan," *Los Angeles Times*, September 30, 1993, accessed September 27, 2025, https://www.latimes.com/archives/la-xpm-1993-09-30-mn-40650-story.html.

53. Erica Jaffe, "Clinton Health Care Reform: The Squandering of Public Support," (paper, Illinois State University Student Conferences, 2005), accessed September 27, 2025, https://pol.illinoisstate.edu/downloads/student-life/conferences/Jaffe2005.pdf.

54. Richard K. Armey and Newt Gingrich, "The Welfarization of Health Care: Clinton Healthcare Reform," *Encyclopedia.com*, February 7, 1994, accessed September 27, 2025, https://www.encyclopedia.com/social-sciences/applied-and-social-sciences-magazines/welfarization-health-care.

55. Paul Starr, "What Happened to Health Care Reform?" *The American Prospect*, no. 20 (Winter 1995): 20–31, accessed September 27, 2025, https://www.princeton.edu/~starr/20starr.html.

56. James Fallows, "A Triumph of Misinformation," *The Atlantic*, January 1995, accessed September 27, 2025, https://www.theatlantic.com/past/politics/healthca/hcfallow.htm.

57. Jaffe, *Clinton Health Care Reform*.

58. Amy Goldstein, "How the Demise of Her Health-Care Plan Led to the Politician Clinton Is Today," *Washington Post*, August 25, 2016, accessed September 27, 2025, https://www.washingtonpost.com/politics/after-health-care-missteps-a-chastened-hillary-clinton-emerged/2016/08/25/2d200cb4-64b4-11e6-be4e-23fc4d4d12b4_story.html.

59. Skocpol, *The Time Is Never Ripe*.

60. Julie Rovner, "Patients' Rights: The Never-Ending Story," *Managed Healthcare Executive*, March 1, 2001, accessed September 27, 2025, https://www.managedhealthcareexecutive.com/view/patients-rights-never-ending-story.

61. Reuters, "Patients' Rights Gets A-OK," *Wired*, August 3, 2001, accessed September 27, 2025, https://www.wired.com/2001/08/patients-rights-gets-a-ok/.

62. Julie Rovner, "Fact Check: Who's Right on Protections for Preexisting Conditions? It's Complicated," *KFF Health News*, October 11, 2018, accessed September 27, 2025, https://kffhealthnews.org/news/fact-check-whos-right-on-protections-for-preexisting-conditions-its-complicated/.

63. "Pre-Existing Conditions Could Affect 1 in 2 Americans," *CMS/CCIIO*, accessed September 27, 2025, https://www.cms.gov/cciio/resources/forms-reports-and-other-resources/preexisting. (cms.gov).

64. "Health Insurance Rights & Protections," HealthCare.gov, accessed September 27, 2025, https://www.healthcare.gov/health-care-law-protections/rights-and-protections/.

65. "Patient Protection and Affordable Care Act; Health Insurance Market Rules; Rate Review," *Federal Register* 78, no. 38 (February 27, 2013): 13406–13435 (to be codified at 45 C.F.R. pts. 144, 147, 150, 154, 156), accessed September 27, 2025, https://www.federalregister.gov/documents/2013/02/27/2013-04335/patient-protection-and-affordable-care-act-health-insurance-market-rules-rate-review.

66. "Cancellations & Appeals," *U.S. Department of Health & Human Services*, accessed September 27, 2025, https://www.hhs.gov/healthcare/about-the-aca/cancellations-and-appeals/index.html. (HHS.gov).

67. "Cancellations & Appeals."

68. Louis Jacobson, "Barack Obama Says That What He'd Said Was You Could Keep Your Plan 'If It Hasn't Changed Since the Law Passed'," *PolitiFact*, November 6, 2013, accessed September 27, 2025, https://www.politifact.com/factchecks/2013/nov/06/barack-obama/barack-obama-says-what-hed-said-was-you-could-keep/.

69. USAFacts Team, "The Affordable Care Act and the Data: Who Is Insured and Who Isn't," *USAFacts*, updated January 17, 2025, accessed September 27, 2025, https://usafacts.org/articles/affordable-care-act-and-data-who-insured-and-who-isnt/.

70. Molly Ball, "How Nancy Pelosi Saved the Affordable Care Act," *TIME*, May 6, 2020, accessed September 27, 2025, https://time.com/5832330/nancy-pelosi-obamacare/.

71. Eric Lutz, "Obama's Memoir Illustrates Why Trump Failed at Destroying the ACA," *Vanity Fair*, October 26, 2020, accessed September 27, 2025, https://www.vanityfair.com/news/2020/10/obama-memoir-promised-land-obamacare-aca.

72. Ball, "How Nancy Pelosi Saved the Affordable Care Act."

73. Ball, "How Nancy Pelosi Saved the Affordable Care Act."

74. Ibid.

75. Ibid.

76. "H.R. 2 – Repealing the Job-Killing Health Care Law Act," *Congress.gov*, 112th Congress, accessed September 27, 2025, https://www.congress.gov/bill/112th-congress/house-bill/2. (congress.gov).

77. John Parkinson, "House Obamacare Repeal: Thirty-Third Time's the Charm?," *ABC News*, July 11, 2012, accessed September 27, 2025, https://abcnews.go.com/blogs/politics/2012/07/house-obamacare-repeal-thirty-third-times-the-charm.

78. "Sen. Ted Cruz Ends 21-Hour Obamacare Filibuster," *New York Post*, September 25, 2013, accessed September 27, 2025, https://nypost.com/2013/09/25/cruz-ends-21-hour-filibuster/.

79. Jonathan Weisman and Ashley Parker, "The President and Congress Face Off Over the Budget," *The New York Times*, October 17, 2013, accessed September 27, 2025, https://www.nytimes.com/2013/10/17/us/congress-budget-debate.html.

80. "Summary of the Restoring Americans' Healthcare Freedom Reconciliation Act of 2015," *Kaiser Family Foundation*, accessed September 27, 2025, https://files.kff.org/attachment/Summary-of-the-Restoring-Americans-Healthcare-Freedom-Reconciliation-Act-of-2015.

81. "Coverage and Premiums in the Health Insurance Marketplaces: CBO's May 2018 Baseline" (Congressional Budget Office, May 2018), accessed September 27, 2025, https://www.cbo.gov/sites/default/files/115th-congress-2017-2018/reports/52371-coverageandpremiums.pdf.

82. Louise Radnofsky, Stephanie Armour, and Anna Wilde Mathews, "Trump to Sign Order Easing Health Plan Rules, Official Says," *Wall Street Journal*, October 7, 2017, accessed September 27, 2025, https://www.wsj.com/articles/trump-to-sign-order-to-expand-health-insurance-options-for-self-insured-1507410483.

83. Evan Saltzman and Christine Eibner, "*Donald Trump's Health Care Reform Proposals: Anticipated Effects on Insurance Coverage, Out-of-Pocket Costs, and the Federal Deficit*" (Issue Brief, September 2016, The Commonwealth Fund), accessed September 27, 2025, https://www.commonwealthfund.org/sites/default/files/documents/___media_files_publications_issue_brief_2016_sep_1903_saltzman_trump_hlt_care_reform_proposals_ib_v2.pdf.

84. @realDonaldTrump, "3 Republicans and 48 Democrats let the American people down. As I said from the beginning, let ObamaCare implode, then deal . . .," *X* (formerly Twitter), July 28, 2017, https://x.com/realDonaldTrump/status/890820505330212864.

85. Peter Jacobs, "John McCain: Here's Why I Voted No," *Yahoo Finance*, July 28, 2017, accessed September 27, 2025, https://finance.yahoo.com/news/john-mccain-heres-why-voted-080525553.html.

86. Burgess Everett and Seung Min Kim, "Why McCain Screwed the GOP on Obamacare Repeal – Again," *Politico*, September 22, 2017, accessed September

27, 2025, https://www.politico.com/story/2017/09/22/john-mccain-obamacare-repeal-opposition-243036.

87. Everett and Kim, "Why McCain Screwed the GOP."

88. "Complaint for Declaratory and Injunctive Relief," U.S. District Court, Northern District of Texas (filed February 26, 2018), in *Affordable Care Act Litigation*, accessed September 27, 2025, https://affordablecareactlitigation.com/wp-content/uploads/2018/09/177111358274.pdf.

89. Ashley Kirzinger, Audrey Kearney, and Mollyann Brodie, "KFF Health Tracking Poll – February 2020: Health Care in the 2020 Election," *Kaiser Family Foundation*, February 21, 2020, accessed September 27, 2025, https://www.kff.org/affordable-care-act/kff-health-tracking-poll-february-2020/.

90. Daniel Cruz and Greg Fann, "It's Not Just the Prices: ACA Plans Have Declined in Quality Over the Past Decade," *Paragon Health Institute*, accessed September 27, 2025, https://paragoninstitute.org/private-health/its-not-just-the-prices-aca-plans-have-declined-in-quality-over-the-past-decade/.

91. Jared Ortaliza, Matt McGough, Cynthia Cox, Kaye Pestaina, Robin Rudowitz, and Alice Burns, "How Will the One Big Beautiful Bill Act Affect the ACA, Medicaid, and the Uninsured Rate?" *Kaiser Family Foundation*, June 18, 2025, accessed September 27, 2025, https://www.kff.org/medicaid/how-will-the-2025-budget-reconciliation-affect-the-aca-medicaid-and-the-uninsured-rate/.

92. Ortaliza et al., "How Will the One Big Beautiful Bill Act Affect the ACA, Medicaid, and the Uninsured Rate?"

93. MoneyGeek, "Average ACA Marketplace Premiums by State, 2026," *MoneyGeek*, updated October 2025, https://www.moneygeek.com/insurance/health/aca-premiums-2026/.

Chapter 3

1. American Brain Tumor Association, "PNET (Primitive Neuroectodermal Tumor)," ABTA, accessed October 13, 2025, https://www.abta.org/tumor_types/pnet/.

2. "Etymology of *Psychosocial*," *Online Etymology Dictionary*, accessed September 24, 2025, https://www.etymonline.com/word/psychosocial.

3. "History of Anesthesia," Wood Library-Museum of Anesthesiology, accessed September 24, 2025, https://www.woodlibrarymuseum.org/history-of-anesthesia/.

4. Betsy Bates, "First FDA-Approved Chemo Agent Turns 60," Internal Medicine News (March 1, 2009), accessed September 24, 2025, https://cdn.mdedge.com/files/s3fs-public/issues/articles/70173_main_4.pdf.

5. Vincent T. DeVita Jr. and Steven A. Rosenberg, "Two Hundred Years of Cancer Research," *New England Journal of Medicine* 366, no. 23 (June 7, 2012): https://www.nejm.org/doi/full/10.1056/NEJMra1204479.

6. American Cancer Society, *Global Cancer Facts & Figures 2025* (Atlanta: American Cancer Society, 2025), PDF, https://www.cancer.org/content/dam/cancer-org/research/cancer-facts-and-statistics/annual-cancer-facts-and-figures/2025/2025-cancer-facts-and-figures-acs.pdf.

7. Emily Tonorezos et al., "Prevalence of Cancer Survivors in the United States," *Journal of the National Cancer Institute* 116, no. 11 (Year): 1784–1790, https://academic.oup.com/jnci/article/116/11/1784/7713374.

Chapter 4

1. Adolescent and Young Adult Oncology Progress Review Group, *Closing the Gap: Research and Care Imperatives for Adolescents and Young Adults with Cancer* (Washington, DC: National Cancer Institute / LIVESTRONG Young Adult Alliance, August 2006), https://www.cancer.gov/types/aya/research/ayao-august-2006.pdf.

2. Carrie Printz, "Adolescent and Young Adult Oncology Comes of Age," *Cancer* 117, no. 24 (December 2, 2011): 5433, https://doi.org/10.1002/cncr.26703.

3. Stupid Cancer (formerly I'm Too Young For This!, i2y), *StupidCancer.com*, archived February 2, 2012, https://web.archive.org/web/20120202121525/http://stupidcancer.com.

4. "OMG Summit 2013," *OMG Summit*, archived September 7, 2012, https://web.archive.org/web/20120907160714/http://omgsummit.org/2013/index.html

5. Charles H. Weaver, "Stupid Cancer." *CancerConnect*, March 8, 2009. https://news.cancerconnect.com/treatment-care/stupid-cancer?

6. "Alli Ward Is a Living Miracle Who Has Defied All the Odds," YouTube video, 21:45, posted by *Stupid Cancer* (June 15, 2017), https://www.youtube.com/watch?v=yCGI2ovptzI.

7. Stupid Cancer, *AYA Patient Bill of Rights*, PDF, accessed September 25, 2025, https://stupidcancer.org/wp-content/uploads/2021/09/AYA-Patient-Bill-of-Rights.pdf.

8. Melinda Beck, "The Wall Street Journal — 'Too Young for Cancer' and Demanding Action," *Friends of Cancer Research*, November 9, 2010, https://friendsofcancerresearch.org/news/the-wall-street-journal-too-young-for-cancer-and-demanding-action/.

9. Jane Sarasohn-Kahn, *The Wisdom of Patients: Health Care Meets Online Social Media* (Oakland, CA: California HealthCare Foundation, April 2008), PDF, accessed July 5, 2025, https://www.chcf.org/wp-content/uploads/2017/12/PDF-HealthCareSocialMedia.pdf.

10. Kenny Kane, "From T-Shirts to Impact: How I Built the Stupid Cancer Store," Kenny Kane (blog), June 2, 2025, https://kenny-kane.com/blog/stupid-cancer-store.

11. Kane, "From T-Shirts to Impact."

12. Manny Alvarez, "Best Health Blogs of 2010," Fox News, December 23, 2010, https://www.foxnews.com/health/best-health-blogs-of-2010.

13. Matthew Zachary, "We Are Stupid Cancer," LinkedIn post, 2018, https://www.linkedin.com/posts/matthewzachary_we-are-stupid-cancer-activity-6382761396764966913-bpZ4.

Chapter 5

1. Adolescent and Young Adult Oncology Progress Review Group, *Closing the Gap: Research and Care Imperatives for Adolescents and Young Adults with Cancer* (Washington, DC: National Cancer Institute / LIVESTRONG Young Adult Alliance, August 2006), https://www.cancer.gov/types/aya/research/ayao-august-2006.pdf.

2. Alba A. Brandes and Enrico Franceschi, "Shedding Light on Adult Medulloblastoma: Current Management and Opportunities for Advances," *ASCO Educational Book* 34 (2014): e82–e87, https://doi.org/10.14694/EdBook_AM.2014.34.e82.

3. "Understanding Hand and Wrist Injuries: A Review on Overuse in Musicians," *Central Health Physiotherapy*, last modified August 12, 2024, https://www.central-health.com/blog/understanding-hand-and-wrist-injuries-a-review-on-overuse-in-musicians/.

4. Matthew Zachary, "The End of Pediatric Cancer Research as We Know It," *U.S. News & World Report*, December 2, 2015, https://health.usnews.com/health-news/patient-advice/articles/2015/12/02/the-end-of-pediatric-cancer-research-as-we-know-it.

5. Matthew Zachary, "The End of Pediatric Cancer Research as We Know It."

6. Bradley Zebrack, "Cancer Survivorship — A Framework for Quality Cancer Care," *Journal of the National Cancer Institute* 116, no. 3 (March 2024): 352, https://academic.oup.com/jnci/article/116/3/352/7479696.

7. "NLM Profiles: Spotlight — Catalog," National Library of Medicine, accessed September 26, 2025, https://profiles.nlm.nih.gov/spotlight/tl/catalog/nlm%3Anlmuid-101584665X20-doc.
8. Judith L. Pearson, *Crusade to Heal America: The Remarkable Life of Mary Lasker* (Rochester, Minn: Mayo Clinic Press, 2023), 182.
9. "Catalyst for the National Cancer Act: Mary Lasker," *Lasker Foundation*, accessed September 26, 2025, https://laskerfoundation.org/catalyst-for-the-national-cancer-act-mary-lasker/.
10. Gabrielle Emanuel, "50 Years Ago, Nixon Gave the U.S. a Christmas Gift: It Launched the 'War on Cancer'," *NPR*, December 23, 2021, accessed September 26, 2025, https://www.npr.org/sections/health-shots/2021/12/23/1058107864/50-years-ago-nixon-gave-the-u-s-a-christmas-gift-it-launched-the-war-on-cancer.
11. Rose Kushner, *Breast Cancer: A Personal History and an Investigative Report* (New York: Harcourt Brace Jovanovich, 1975), 15.
12. Barron Lerner, "No Shrinking Violet: Rose Kushner and the Rise of American Breast Cancer Activism," *Western Journal of Medicine* 174, no. 5 (May 2001): 362–65, https://www.ncbi.nlm.nih.gov/pmc/articles/PMC1071404/.
13. National Coalition for Cancer Survivorship, *Seasons of Survival* (Washington, DC: National Coalition for Cancer Survivorship, 2013), accessed September 26, 2025, https://canceradvocacy.org/wp-content/uploads/2013/01/Seasons-of-Survival.pdf.
14. Ibid.
15. Ibid.
16. Cancer History Project, "Harold Freeman, Father of Patient Navigation, on Cutting the Cancer out of Harlem," *Cancer History Project*, February 11, 2022, accessed September 26, 2025, https://cancerhistoryproject.com/people/harold-freeman-cutting-cancer-out-of-harlem/.
17. National Coalition for Cancer Survivorship, *Imperatives for Quality Cancer Care: Access, Advocacy, Action, and Accountability* (Silver Spring, MD: National Coalition for Cancer Survivorship, 1996), accessed September 26, 2025, https://canceradvocacy.org/wp-content/uploads/2013/01/NCCS_Imperatives_8-96.pdf.
18. Cancer History Project, "A Biography of the Cancer Survivorship Movement: The March," *The Cancer History Project*, March 11, 2021, https://cancerhistoryproject.com/article/a-biography-of-the-cancer-survivorship-movement-the-march, accessed September 26, 2025, https://cancerhistoryproject.com/article/a-biography-of-the-cancer-survivorship-movement-the-march/.
19. Amy Argetsinger and Craig Whitlock, "Thousands March to Spur Cancer Research," *Washington Post*, September 26, 1998, https://www.washingtonpost

.com/archive/politics/1998/09/27/thousands-march-to-spur-cancer-research/
478c196c-b07a-4104-ae5a-5e3fdef4bb18/.

20. American Cancer Society, *Cancer Facts & Figures 2005* (Atlanta: American Cancer Society, 2005), https://www.cancer.org/content/dam/cancer-org/research/cancer-facts-and-statistics/annual-cancer-facts-and-figures/2005/cancer-facts-and-figures-2005.pdf.

21. Matthew Zachary, "EP4: You're Not 'Cured' – You're Just Not Dead," *The Cancer Mavericks: A History of Survivorship*, September 10, 2021, accessed October 3, 2025, https://www.podpage.com/cancermavericks/im-alive-help/.

22. Committee on Cancer Survivorship, *"From Cancer Patient to Cancer Survivor: Lost in Transition,"* ed. Maria Hewitt, Sheldon Greenfield, and Ellen Stovall (Washington, DC: National Academies Press, 2006), accessed September 26, 2025, https://www.georgiacancerinfo.org/articleImages/articlePDF_396.pdf.

23. UCLA Health, "UCLA Jonsson Cancer Center Named a Survivorship Center of Excellence," March 26, 2006, https://www.uclahealth.org/news/release/ucla-jonsson-cancer-center-named-survivorship-center.

24. "Beyond Survival," *Cancer Today*, Fall 2013, 28, accessed September 26, 2025, https://www.cancertoday-digital.org/cancertoday/fall_2013?pg=28#pg28.

25. Matthew Zachary, "EP5: The Young Adult Cancer Revolution: When the Next Generation Got Loud," *The Cancer Mavericks: A History of Survivorship*, October 8, 2021, accessed October 3, 2025, https://www.podpage.com/cancermavericks/the-young-adult-cancer-movement/.

26. Zachary, "The Young Adult Cancer Revolution."

27. Emily McCullar, "Making the Band: An Oral History of the LIVESTRONG Bracelet," *Texas Monthly*, July 2024, PDF, https://LIVESTRONG.org/wp-content/uploads/2024/07/TM_0724_LIVESTRONG.pdf.

28. Nicole Cobler and Asher Price, "Iconic LIVESTRONG Bracelet Turns 20 Years Old," *Axios Austin*, August 7, 2024, accessed September 27, 2025, https://www.axios.com/local/austin/2024/08/07/iconic-LIVESTRONG-bracelet-turns-20-years-old.

29. "Katie Couric Gets a Colonoscopy," *Today Show* video, 9:59 March 7, 2000, NBC News, https://www.today.com/video/katie-couric-gets-a-colonoscopy-1191167555989.

30. Stand Up To Cancer, *"SU2C Fact Sheet / Overview"* January 4, 2024," PDF (Stand Up To Cancer), accessed September 27, 2025, https://news.standuptocancer.org/wp-content/uploads/SU2C-Fact-Sheet-Overview_01.04.2024.pdf.

31. U.S. Government Accountability Office, "Indian Health Service: Spending Levels and Characteristics of IHS and Three Other Federal Health Care

Programs," GAO-19-74R, December 10, 2018, accessed September 27, 2025, https://www.gao.gov/products/gao-19-74r.

32. Matthew Zachary, "EP7: The Inequity of Cure: Who Gets to Matter," *The Cancer Mavericks: A History of Survivorship*, December 17, 2021, accessed October 3, 2025, https://www.podpage.com/cancermavericks/cancer-doesnt-suck-equally/.

Chapter 6

1. Kris Carr, "Reclaim Your Life — Even with Cancer," *KrisCarr.com*, accessed September 28, 2025, https://kriscarr.com/get/your-cancer-guide/.

2. Louise Norris, "HMO vs PPO vs POS vs EPO: What's the Difference?," *Health Insurance.org*, February 17, 2025, https://www.healthinsurance.org/blog/hmo-ppo-epo-or-pos-choosing-a-managed-care-option/.

3. Jordyn Bradley, "What Medicaid Recipients Should Know About the 'One Big Beautiful Bill,'" *Investopedia*, July 20, 2025, https://www.investopedia.com/what-medicaid-recipients-should-know-about-the-one-big-beautiful-bill-11773484.

4. American Academy of Pediatrics, "AAP Analysis: 49 % of Children Insured by Medicaid or CHIP," *AAP News*, February 27, 2025, https://publications.aap.org/aapnews/news/31491/AAP-analysis-49-of-children-insured-by-Medicaid-or.

5. Marshall Allen, *Never Pay the First Bill: And Other Ways to Fight the Health Care System and Win* (New York: Portfolio, 2021), 48.

6. Mike Kroupa, "Self-Funded Insurance vs Fully Insured," *CGO on the Go Blog*, accessed September 28, 2025, https://www.gocgo.com/blog/self-funded-insurance-vs-fully-insured.

7. Tanya Albert Henry, "Over 80% of Prior Auth Appeals Succeed. Why Aren't There More?," *AMA (American Medical Association)*, October 3, 2024, https://www.ama-assn.org/practice-management/prior-authorization/over-80-prior-auth-appeals-succeed-why-aren-t-there-more.

8. Justin Lo, Michelle Long, Rayna Wallace, Meghan Salaga, and Kaye Pestaina, "Claims Denials and Appeals in ACA Marketplace Plans in 2023," *KFF*, January 27, 2025, accessed September 27, 2025, https://www.kff.org/private-insurance/claims-denials-and-appeals-in-aca-marketplace-plans-in-2023/. (kff.org).

9. Ashley Valentino, "What to Do if Health Insurance Denies a Prior Authorization for Treatment," *Keck Medicine of USC Blog*, last updated May 8, 2025, https://www.keckmedicine.org/blog/health-insurance-claims/.

10. "Internal appeals," *HealthCare.gov*, accessed September 28, 2025, https://www.healthcare.gov/appeal-insurance-company-decision/internal-appeals/.

11. "Guidance on External Review for Group Health Plans and Health Insurance Issuers" (Technical Release 2011-02), U.S. Department of Health & Human Services / CMS, June 22, 2011, https://www.cms.gov/CCIIO/Resources/Files/Downloads/appeals_srg_update.pdf.

12. Stephanie Guinan, "Insurance Claim Denials: Worst Companies and How to Appeal," *ValuePenguin*, May 15, 2024, https://www.valuepenguin.com/health-insurance-claim-denials-and-appeals. (American Economic Liberties Project).

13. "Patients Are Using AI to Fight Insurance Denials," *Winsome Marketing*, July 22, 2025, https://winsomemarketing.com/ai-in-marketing/patients-are-using-ai-to-fight-insurance-denials.

14. Consumer Financial Protection Bureau, *Medical Debt Burden in the United States*, February 2022, https://files.consumerfinance.gov/f/documents/cfpb_medical-debt-burden-in-the-united-states_report_2022-03.pdf.

15. "The One Big Beautiful Bill Act (OBBBA) & Credit Reporting Rule — What You Need to Know," *Undue Medical Debt*, July 25, 2025, https://unduemedicaldebt.org/the-one-big-beautiful-bill-act-obbba-credit-reporting-rule-what-you-need-to-know/.

16. David Kendall, Blair Elliott & Timothy Kusuma, "GOP Health Care Cuts: A Recipe for Medical Debt Disaster," *Third Way*, June 23, 2025, updated September 9, 2025, https://www.thirdway.org/memo/gop-health-care-cuts-a-recipe-for-medical-debt-disaster.

17. "The Most Expensive Medical Diseases and Procedures," USC Price School *Price Blog*, November 17, 2023. https://priceschool.usc.edu/price-blog/the-most-expensive-medical-diseases-and-procedures/ (priceschool.usc.edu)

18. Brianna Abbott and Peter Loftus, "Cancer Is Capsizing Americans' Finances. 'I Was Losing Everything,'" *Wall Street Journal*, May 28, 2024, https://www.wsj.com/health/healthcare/cancer-cost-patient-debt-dd7c540c.

19. Nich Tremper, "Behind the Boom in Solopreneurship: Who's Starting Them and Why," *Gusto Insights*, July 31, 2025, https://gusto.com/resources/gusto-insights/new-business-formation-solopreneurs-2025.

20. Joseph M. Unger, "Inclusive Cancer Clinical Trial Participation—A Recipe for New Treatment Advances," *JAMA Network Open* 8, no. 6 (June 12, 2025): e2515210, https://doi.org/10.1001/jamanetworkopen.2025.15210.

21. Joseph M. Unger, Lawrence N. Shulman, Matthew A. Facktor, Heidi Nelson, and Mark E. Fleury, "National Estimates of the Participation of Patients with

Cancer in Clinical Research Studies Based on Commission on Cancer Accreditation Data," *Journal of Clinical Oncology* 42, no. 18 (June, 2024): 2139–2148, https://doi.org/10.1200/JCO.23.01030.

22. Lauren M. Hamel, Louis A. Penner, Terrance L. Albrecht, Elisabeth Heath, Clement K. Gwede, and Susan Eggly, "Barriers to Clinical Trial Enrollment in Racial and Ethnic Minority Patients with Cancer," *Cancer Control* 23, no. 4 (October 2016): 327–337, https://www.ncbi.nlm.nih.gov/pmc/articles/PMC5131730/.

23. *National Cancer Institute*, "Who Pays for Clinical Trials?" updated November 7, 2024, National Institutes of Health. See https://www.cancer.gov/research/participate/clinical-trials/paying.

Chapter 7

1. Luke Darby, "Jon Stewart Tore into Congress Over 9/11 First Responders' Fund," *GQ*, June 12, 2019, accessed September 27, 2025, https://www.gq.com/story/jon-stewart-congress-first-responders.

2. "H.R. 1,327 – Never Forget the Heroes: James Zadroga, Ray Pfeifer, and Luis Alvarez Permanent Authorization of the September 11th Victim Compensation Fund Act," *Congress.gov*, 116th Congress, accessed September 27, 2025, https://www.congress.gov/bill/116th-congress/house-bill/1327.

3. "Jon Stewart's Entire Testimony Before Congress for 9/11 First Responders," YouTube video, duration n.d., posted by *New York Post*, accessed September 27, 2025, https://www.youtube.com/watch?v=WdRGL2ET2i0.

4. "Jon Stewart's Entire Testimony Before Congress for 9/11 First Responders."

5. Emily Tillett and Grace Segers, "Jon Stewart Lashes Out at House Panel over 9/11 Victim Compensation Fund: 'You Should Be Ashamed of Yourselves'," *CBS News*, June 11, 2019, accessed September 27, 2025, https://www.cbsnews.com/news/victim-compensation-fund-jon-stewart-lashes-out-at-house-hearing-on-911-responders-bill-you-should-be-ashamed-of/.

6. "Jon Stewart's Entire Testimony Before Congress for 9/11 First Responders."

7. Devlin Barrett, "9/11 Victims Bill Stalls as Republican Senators Seek Conditions for Funding," *Washington Post*, July 17, 2019, accessed September 27, 2025, https://www.washingtonpost.com/national-security/two-republican-senators-emerge-as-opponents-to-911-victims-bill/2019/07/17/b6fe830a-a89c-11e9-86dd-d7f0e60391e9_story.html.

8. "Attempted Cuts to the Staff of the World Trade Center Health Program and Cuts to 9–11 Cancer Research," *Renew911Health.org*, accessed September 27, 2025, https://www.renew911health.org/attempted-cuts-to-the-staff-of-the-world-trade-center-health-program-and-cuts-to-9-11-cancer-research/.

9. National Coalition for Cancer Survivorship, *NCCS* 2, no. 4 (Fall 1988), https://cdn.cancerhistoryproject.com/media/2021/04/12170838/NCCS-2-4-Fall-1988.pdf.

10. Hearing on Discrimination Against Cancer Victims and the Handicapped: Hearing Before the Subcommittee on Employment Opportunities of the Committee on Education and Labor, House of Representatives, One Hundredth Congress, *First Session, June 17, 1987*, Serial No. 100–31 (Washington, DC: U.S. Government Printing Office, 1987), https://files.eric.ed.gov/fulltext/ED306749.pdf.

11. Larry Levitt, Anthony Damico, Gary Claxton, Cynthia Cox, and Karen Pollitz, *Gaps in Coverage Among People With Pre-Existing Conditions* (issue brief, Kaiser Family Foundation, May 17, 2017), https://www.kff.org/affordable-care-act/issue-brief/gaps-in-coverage-among-people-with-pre-existing-conditions/.

12. National Coalition for Cancer Survivorship (NCCS), "NCCS Statement on the American Health Care Act," March 7, 2017, CancerAdvocacy, https://cancerad vocacy.org/nccs-statement-american-health-care-act/.

13. National Coalition for Cancer Survivorship, "NCCS Statement on the American Health Care Act."

14. Abby Curtis, "Flap Reconstruction Surgery (Autologous Reconstruction)," *Breastcancer.org*, last updated August 31, 2024, https://www.breastcancer.org/treatment/surgery/breast-reconstruction/types/autologous-flap.

15. Jen Uscher, "DIEP Flap Reconstruction Procedure," *Breastcancer.org*, last updated April 29, 2025, https://www.breastcancer.org/treatment/surgery/breast-reconstruction/types/autologous-flap/diep.

16. Claragh Healy and Robert J. Allen Sr., "The Evolution of Perforator Flap Breast Reconstruction: Twenty Years after the First DIEP Flap," *Journal of Reconstructive Microsurgery* 30, no. 2 (2014): 121–126, https://www.thieme-connect.com/products/ejournals/html/10.1055/s-0033-1357272.

17. Rachana Pradhan, Anna Werner, and Leigh Ann Winick, "After Backlash, Feds Cancel Plan That Risked Limiting Breast Reconstruction Options," *KFF Health News*, August 23, 2023, https://kffhealthnews.org/news/article/cms-ruling-diep-flap-breast-reconstruction/.

18. Centers for Medicare & Medicaid Services, *2021 HCPCS Application Summary: Second Biannual, Non-Drug and Non-Biological Items and Services* (Baltimore, MD: CMS, 2021), https://www.cms.gov/files/document/2021-hcpcs-application-summary-biannual-2-2021-non-drug-and-non-biological-items-and-services.pdf.

19. Pradhan, Werner, and Winick, "After Backlash, Feds Cancel Plan That Risked Limiting Breast Reconstruction Options."

20. National Coalition for Cancer Survivorship (NCCS), "NCCS Urges CMS to Preserve Access to DIEP Flap Breast Reconstruction," Cancer Nation, June 1, 2023, https://canceradvocacy.org/nccs-urges-cms-preserve-access-diep-flap-breast-reconstruction/.

21. Lisa D. T. Rice, "CMS Must Protect Access to the 'Gold Standard of Breast Reconstruction'," STAT, June 30, 2023, https://www.statnews.com/2023/06/30/diep-flap-surgery-breast-reconstruction-cancer/.

22. Karen Pollitz, "No Surprises Act Implementation: What to Expect in 2022," KFF, December 10, 2021, accessed September 28, 2025, https://www.kff.org/report-section/no-surprises-act-implementation-what-to-expect-in-2022-appendices.

23. Senator Maggie Hassan, "Senator Hassan to Host Donna Beckman, Who Faced a Surprise Medical Bill, as Her State of the Union Guest," press release, January 31, 2019, https://www.hassan.senate.gov/news/press-releases/senator-hassan-to-host-donna-beckman-who-faced-a-surprise-medical-bill-as-her-state-of-the-union-guest.

24. Ashley Kirzinger, Bryan Wu, Cailey Muñana, and Mollyann Brodie, "Kaiser Health Tracking Poll – Late Summer 2018: The Election, Pre-Existing Conditions, and Surprises on Medical Bills," Kaiser Family Foundation, September 5, 2018, https://www.kff.org/health-costs/poll-finding/kaiser-health-tracking-poll-late-summer-2018-the-election-pre-existing-conditions-and-surprises-on-medical-bills/.

25. Rachel Bluth and Emmarie Huetteman, "Equity Firms and Venture Capitalists Lobby to Save Surprise Medical Bills," Truthout, September 12, 2019, https://truthout.org/articles/equity-firms-and-venture-capitalists-lobby-to-save-surprise-medical-bills/.

26. "Envision Healthcare to be Acquired by KKR for $46.00 Per Share in All-Cash Transaction," Exhibit 99.1, filing of Envision Healthcare Corporation, June 11, 2018, SEC, https://www.sec.gov/Archives/edgar/data/1678531/000119312518188699/d606502dex991.htm.

27. Christina Caron, "Families Fight Back Against Surprise Air Ambulance Bills," The New York Times, April 17, 2020, https://www.nytimes.com/2020/04/17/parenting/air-ambulance-bills.html.

28. Caron, "Families Fight Back Against Surprise Air Ambulance Bills."

29. Mary Bugbee, "Envision Healthcare: A Private Equity Case Study," Private Equity Stakeholder Project, December 2022, 4, https://pestakeholder.org/wp-content/uploads/2022/12/Envision_CaseStudy_Final_Dec2022.pdf.

30. Robert C. "Bobby" Scott and Virginia Foxx, "Congress Protected Patients by Banning Surprise Bills – Attempts to Weaken the Law Shouldn't Stand," The

Hill, April 11, 2022, accessed September 28, 2025, https://thehill.com/blogs/congress-blog/3263784-congress-protected-patients-by-banning-surprise-bills-attempts-to-weaken-the-law-shouldnt-stand/.

31. Bill Cassidy and Maggie Hassan, "Cassidy, Hassan Legislation Ending Surprise Medical Bills Goes into Effect Today," press release, January 1, 2022, https://www.cassidy.senate.gov/newsroom/press-releases/cassidy-hassan-legislation-ending-surprise-medical-bills-goes-into-effect-today/.

32. T. Christian Miller, "Some Surprises in the No Surprises Act," ProPublica, June 28, 2024, https://www.propublica.org/article/no-surprises-act-health-insurance-premiums-doctors-health-care.

33. Miller, "Some Surprises in the No Surprises Act."

34. Rebecca Pifer, "More than One-Fifth of Insurers Failed to Pay No Surprises Awards Last Year, Provider Lobby Says," *Healthcare Dive*, August 28, 2024, https://www.healthcaredive.com/news/more-one-fifth-of-insurers-failed-pay-no-surprises-awards-last-year-providers/725482/.

35. Sydney Halleman, "Envision Healthcare Files for Chapter 11 Bankruptcy," *Healthcare Dive*, May 15, 2023, https://www.healthcaredive.com/news/envision-chapter-11-bankruptcy/650277/.

36. *Cancer Screening, Treatment, and Survivorship Act of 2007*, S. 1415, 110th Cong., https://www.govinfo.gov/content/pkg/BILLS-110s1415is/html/BILLS-110s1415is.htm.

37. Erin Zammet Ruddy, "Today Is LIVESTRONG Day," *Glamour*, May 16, 2007, https://www.glamour.com/story/today-is-LIVESTRONG-day.

38. "Lance Armstrong, Senator Harkin, Senator Snowe, Representative Schakowsky and Representative Myrick Urge Support for the Cancer Screening, Treatment, and Survivorship Act of 2007," *Chron* (Houston), May 17, 2007, https://www.chron.com/news/article/prn-lance-armstrong-senator-harkin-senator-1794862.php.

39. "Preventive Services Covered by Private Health Plans Under the Affordable Care Act," fact sheet, KFF, February 28, 2024, https://www.kff.org/womens-health-policy/preventive-services-covered-by-private-health-plans/.

40. Bill Gifford, "It's Not About the Lab Rats," *Outside Online*, January 5, 2012, https://www.outsideonline.com/outdoor-adventure/biking/its-not-about-lab-rats/.

41. Christi Ball Loso, "Survivorship Program Leads Nationwide Study," Fred Hutch, April 5, 2013, https://www.fredhutch.org/en/news/center-news/2013/04/survivorship-program-leads-nationwide-study.html.

42. Marci K. Campbell et al., "Adult Cancer Survivorship Care: Experiences from the LIVESTRONG Centers of Excellence Network," *Journal of Cancer*

Survivorship 5, no. 3 (2011 May 10): 271–282, https://doi.org/10.1007/s11764-011-0180-z, https://www.ncbi.nlm.nih.gov/pmc/articles/PMC3739450/

43. Academy of Oncology Nurse & Patient Navigators (AONN+), "Oncology Navigation Standards of Professional Practice, *Journal of Oncology Navigation & Survivorship*," March 2022, https://d2geqc87xuuo99.cloudfront.net/pdf/2022/jons/0322_JONS_PONT.pdf.

44. Oncology Nursing Society, "Role of the Oncology Nurse Navigator Throughout the Cancer Trajectory," position statement, accessed September 28, 2025, https://www.ons.org/network-advocacy/position-statements/role-oncology-nurse-navigator-throughout-cancer-trajectory.

45. U.S. Government Accountability Office, "Breast Cancer Education: HHS Has Implemented Initiatives Aimed at Young Women," GAO-17-19 December 2016, https://www.gao.gov/assets/gao-17-19.pdf.

46. Rep. Debbie Wasserman Schultz, "Breast Cancer," *U.S. House of Representatives*, accessed September 28, 2025, https://wassermanschultz.house.gov/issues/issue/?IssueID=15060.

47. Prevent Cancer Foundation, "Prevent Cancer Foundation Responds to New Breast Cancer Screening Guidelines Issued by the U.S. Preventive Services Task Force," April 30, 2024, accessed September 28, 2025, https://preventcancer.org/news/prevent-cancer-foundation-responds-to-new-breast-cancer-screening-guidelines-issued-by-the-u-s-preventive-services-task-force/.

48. "MDSave," *Lumbar Spine Fusion (Inpatient)*, accessed September 28, 2025, https://tinyurl.com/ebhbpdef.

49. Kaiser Family Foundation, *Individual Market Guaranteed Issue (Not Applicable to HIPAA-Eligible Individuals)*, accessed September 28, 2025, https://www.kff.org/state-health-policy-data/state-indicator/individual-market-guaranteed-issue-not-applicable-to-hipaa-eligible-individuals

50. MaryBeth Musumeci, *Explaining California v. Texas: A Guide to the Case Challenging the ACA* (issue brief, KFF, September 1, 2020), https://www.kff.org/affordable-care-act/explaining-california-v-texas-a-guide-to-the-case-challenging-the-aca/.

51. Julie Rovner, "Fact Check: Who's Right on Protections for Preexisting Conditions? It's Complicated," *KFF Health News*, October 11, 2018, https://kffhealthnews.org/news/fact-check-whos-right-on-protections-for-preexisting-conditions-its-complicated/.

52. Jacob Gardenswartz, "Biden's on Target About What Repealing ACA Would Mean for Preexisting Condition Protections," *KFF Health News*, June 13, 2024, https://kffhealthnews.org/news/article/fact-check-biden-campaign-ad-repealing-obamacare-preexisting-conditions/.

53. Maanasa Kona and Sabrina Corlette, "State Efforts to Protect Preexisting Conditions Unsustainable Without the ACA," *To the Point* (blog), Commonwealth Fund, October 29, 2020, https://www.commonwealthfund.org/blog/2020/state-efforts-preexisting-conditions.

54. Kaiser Family Foundation, "Individual Market Guaranteed Issue (Not Applicable to HIPAA-Eligible Individuals," accessed September 28, 2025, https://www.kff.org/other/state-indicator/individual-market-guaranteed-issue-not-applicable-to-hipaa-eligible-individuals/.

55. "Health Insurance Reform in the 1990s: A Kentucky Historical Perspective," Kentucky Department of Insurance, https://insurance.ky.gov/ppc/Documents/history.pdf.

56. "Challenges of Partial Reform – Lessons from State Efforts to Reform the Individual and Small group Market before the Affordable Care" PWC, February, 2017), https://www.chcf.org/wp-content/uploads/2017/12/PDF-ChallengesStateReformBeforeACA.pdf.

57. Bruce Schreiner and Dylan Lovan, "Former Kentucky Gov. Brereton Jones Dies, Fought to Bolster Health Care and Ethics Laws in Office," *AP News*, September 18, 2023. https://apnews.com/article/e155dcb44af77ed784d2e14d8214d94f.

58. "A Guide To Repealing ObamaCare, Hidden In Plain Sight" *Investor's Business Daily*, April 13, 2017, accessed September 28, 2025, https://www.investors.com/politics/editorials/a-guide-to-repealing-obamacare-hidden-in-plain-site/.

59. Cynthia Cox, "Back to the Future? A Look Back at High-Risk Pools," *KFF QuickTake*, September 20, 2024, https://www.kff.org/quick-take/back-to-the-future-a-look-back-at-high-risk-pools/.

60. Gary Claxton, Cynthia Cox, Anthony Damico, Larry Levitt, and Karen Pollitz, "Pre-existing Conditions and Medical Underwriting in the Individual Insurance Market Prior to the ACA" (San Francisco: Kaiser Family Foundation, December 12, 2016), https://www.kff.org/private-insurance/pre-existing-conditions-and-medical-underwriting-in-the-individual-insurance-market-prior-to-the-aca/.

61. John E. McDonough, "Mad About States," *Milbank Quarterly*, March 2018, https://www.milbank.org/quarterly/articles/mad-about-states/. (milbank.org).

62. McDonough, "Mad About States."

63. Adriana Morga and Cora Lewis, "Federal Judge Reverses Rule That Would Have Removed Medical Debt from Credit Reports," Associated Press, July 15, 2025, https://apnews.com/article/cfpb-medical-debt-credit-reports-41f212ee6b89f9902deb267d75ab8443.

64. National Consumer Law Center, "Trump Administration Tries to Block State Safeguards from Damaging Medical Debt on Credit Reports," October 30, 2025,

https://www.nclc.org/trump-administration-tries-to-block-state-safeguards-from-damaging-medical-debt-on-credit-reports/.

65. Sarah Kliff and Josh Katz, "Hospitals and Insurers Didn't Want You to See These Prices. Here's Why," *The New York Times*, August 22, 2021, https://www.nytimes.com/interactive/2021/08/22/upshot/hospital-prices.html.

66. "Improving Price and Quality Transparency in American Healthcare to Put Patients First," Proposed Rule, *Federal Register*, June 27, 2019, https://www.federalregister.gov/documents/2019/06/27/2019-13945/improving-price-and-quality-transparency-in-american-healthcare-to-put-patients-first.

67. Chris Smith, Joseph Boschert, Mike Gaal, and David Lewis, "Hospital Price Transparency: December 2021 Update," *Milliman Insight*, December 10, 2021, https://www.milliman.com/en/insight/hospital-price-transparency-december-2021-update.

68. John Kennedy, "Hospitals Can't Keep Hiding Their Prices from Patients," *National Review* (reprinted on the U.S. Senate John Kennedy site), July 17, 2025, https://www.kennedy.senate.gov/public/op-eds?ID=C5C02478-ACAF-4787-A32A-989974F17925.

69. Daniel J. Cognetti, "Editorial Commentary: Hospital Price Transparency Is Neither Patient-Centric Nor Fully Compliant," *Arthroscopy* 41, no. 1 (2025): 128–129, https://pubmed.ncbi.nlm.nih.gov/38830437/.

70. Jade Gomez, "Fat Joe Pushes for Healthcare Price Transparency in New Power to the Patients PSA," *People*, October 3, 2024, https://people.com/fat-joe-pushes-for-healthcare-price-transparency-in-new-power-to-the-patients-psa-8722564.

71. Senator John Kennedy, tweet, July 17, 2025, https://x.com/SenJohnKennedy/status/1945923484741165310.

72. Patient Rights Advocate, "New Poll: An Unparalleled 96% of Americans Support Healthcare Price Transparency," May 20, 2025, accessed September 28, 2025, https://www.patientrightsadvocate.org/blog/new-poll-an-unparalleled-96-of-americans-support-healthcare-price-transparency.

73. *Dollar For, Bridging the Chasm* (April 2024), https://dollarfor.org/wp-content/uploads/2024/04/Dollar_For.Bridging_the_Chasm.pdf.

74. Anna Wilde Mathews, Andrea Fuller, and Melanie Evans, "Hospitals Often Don't Help Needy Patients, Even Those Who Qualify," *Wall Street Journal*, November 17, 2022, https://www.wsj.com/articles/nonprofit-hospitals-financial-aid-charity-care-11668696836.

75. *Dollar For, Fixing Hospital Financial Assistance: A One-Pager* (2025), https://dollarfor.org/wp-content/uploads/2025/05/fixing_hfa_1pager.pdf.

76. Dollar For, "Impact Numbers," accessed September 28, 2025, https://dollarfor
.org/impact-numbers/.

77. Texas House Bill 3708, 89th Leg., R.S. (2025), *An Act Relating to Charity Care Provided by Certain Health Care Facilities*, Texas Legislature Online,
accessed January 16, 2026, https://capitol.texas.gov/tlodocs/89R/billtext/html/
HB03708I.htm.

78. Christy Snodgrass, LinkedIn post, The Dollar For team was up past midnight
testifying at the Texas Capitol on HB3708 . . ., May 2025, LinkedIn, accessed
January 16, 2026, https://www.linkedin.com/posts/christysnodgrass_the-dollar-
for-team-was-up-past-midnight-activity-7323736901633433600-_9xW/.

79. Kaiser Family Foundation, *KFF Health Care Debt Survey: Main Findings*,
accessed September 28, 2025, https://www.kff.org/report-section/kff-health-
care-debt-survey-main-findings/.

80. Kaiser Family Foundation, *KFF Health Care Debt Survey: Main Findings*.

81. National Consumer Law Center, *Model Law: Medical Debt*, March 2025,
https://www.nclc.org/wp-content/uploads/2022/08/2025.03_Model-Law_
Medical-Debt.pdf.

82. National Consumer Law Center, *Model Law: Medical Debt*.

83. Health Care for All Oregon, "Task Force (JTFUHC) – Oregon's Joint Task
Force on Universal Health Care," accessed September 28, 2025, https://www
.hcao.org/task-force-jtfuhc.

84. Health Care for All Oregon, "Learn," accessed September 28, 2025, https://
www.hcao.org/learn.

85. Health Care for All Oregon, "Legislation," accessed September 28, 2025,
https://www.hcao.org/legislation.

86. Health Care for All Oregon, "Path to Single Payer," accessed September 28,
2025, https://www.hcao.org/path-to-single-payer.

87. Peter Hirschfeld, "Shumlin: It's 'Not the Right Time' for Single Payer," *Vermont
Public*, December 17, 2014, https://www.vermontpublic.org/vpr-news/2014-
12-17/shumlin-its-not-the-right-time-for-single-payer.

88. Angela Hart, "The Demise of Single-Payer in California Trips Up Efforts in
Other States," *The Lund Report*, March 1, 2022, https://www.thelundreport.org/
content/demise-single-payer-california-trips-efforts-other-states.

89. Tobias Coughlin-Bogue, "We Could Have Had Universal Healthcare," *The Stran
ger*, March 17, 2025, https://www.thestranger.com/news/2025/03/17/79971060/
we-could-have-had-universal-healthcare.

90. Zain Khawaja and Ammar Kazi "It's High Time States Banned PBM-Owned
Pharmacies," *MedPage Today*, August 17, 2025, https://www.medpagetoday
.com/opinion/second-opinions/117028?xid=nl_mpt_DHE_2025-08-17.

91. Amanda Rachidi, "PBM Reform Takes Off in 2025," *Pharmacy Times*, April 11, 2025, https://www.pharmacytimes.com/view/pbm-reform-takes-off-in-2025.

92. E. Michael Murphy, "The Year of PBM Reform: Pharmacy Policy Progress Across the States in 2025," *Pharmacist*, July 16, 2025, https://www.pharmacist.com/Blogs/Voices-of-APhA/Article/the-year-of-pbm-reform-pharmacy-policy-progress-across-the-states-in-2025.

Chapter 8

1. Regan Brumagen, "Unsafe at Any Speed," *Encyclopædia Britannica*, accessed October 5, 2025, https://www.britannica.com/topic/Unsafe-at-Any-Speed.

2. Richard Weingroff, "A Moment in Time: Highway Safety Breakthrough," *Federal Highway Administration*, U.S. Department of Transportation, accessed October 5, 2025, https://highways.dot.gov/highway-history/general-highway-history/moment-time-highway-safety-breakthrough.

3. Ibid.

4. "Ralph Nader Reflects On His Auto Safety Campaign, 55 Years Later," *Science Friday*, accessed October 5, 2025, https://www.sciencefriday.com/segments/ralph-nader-auto-safety/.

5. HISTORY.com Editors, "Auto Safety Crusader Ralph Nader Testifies Before Congress," *History*, last updated May 27, 2025, accessed October 5, 2025, https://www.history.com/this-day-in-history/auto-safety-crusader-ralph-nader-testifies-before-congress.

6. "Report Crappy Funders," *Nonprofit AF*, accessed October 5, 2025, https://nonprofitaf.com/report-crappy-funders/.

7. "Overhead: Dan Pallotta on How Great Nonprofits Actually Work" – *Out of Patients with Matthew Zachary* (podcasts.apple.com).

8. Nina Agrawal, "Pediatric Brain Cancer Group to Lose Federal Funding," *The New York Times*, August 28, 2025, accessed October 5, 2025, https://www.nytimes.com/2025/08/28/well/pediatric-brain-cancer-trial-group.html.

9. Michael Sainato, "Cancer Experts Alarmed Over 'Gut-Wrenching' Trump Plan to Cut Research Spending by Billions," *The Guardian*, June 26, 2025, accessed October 4, 2025, https://www.theguardian.com/us-news/2025/jun/26/cancer-research-trump-nci-cuts-plan.

10. Lauran Neergaard and Michael Casey, "Judge Extends Temporary Block to Huge Cuts in National Institutes of Health Research Funding," *AP News*, February 21, 2025, accessed October 5, 2025, https://apnews.com/article/

trump-nih-medical-research-funding-cut-indirect-costs-a75b8d7d56a29f1e88
0859d79ef744e4.

11. Shefali Luthra, "A Promising Path to Breast Cancer Treatment Just Hit a Road-block," *19th News*, August 7, 2025, accessed October 5, 2025, https://19thnews
.org/2025/08/mrna-funding-cuts-cancer-research/.

12. Fumiko Chino, "Cuts to Cancer Research Can't Diminish Hope," STAT, August 6, 2025, accessed October 5, 2025, https://www.statnews.com/2025/08/06/
cancer-research-cuts-nih-budget-hope/.

13. Nicole Leonard, "Pennsylvania Cancer Survivors, Doctors Say Proposed Cuts to Federal Funding Could Delay Breakthroughs," *WHYY*, August 27, 2025, accessed October 5, 2025, https://whyy.org/articles/pennsylvania-cancer-advocates-research-cuts/.

14. Matt Bruenig, "Health Care Administration Wastes Half a Trillion Dollars Every Year," *People's Policy Project*, December 10, 2024, accessed October 5, 2025, https://www.peoplespolicyproject.org/2024/12/10/health-care-administration-wastes-half-a-trillion-dollars-every-year/.

15. Christopher Ingraham, "A Man Radicalized by Statistics," *Pennsylvania Capital-Star*, December 12, 2024, accessed October 5, 2025, https://penncapital-star
.com/criminal-justice/mangione-a-man-radicalized-by-statistics/.

16. Ibid.

17. "Buffett's Berkshire Acquires 5 Million Shares in UnitedHealth," *Reuters*, August 14, 2025, accessed October 5, 2025, https://www.reuters.com/business/
healthcare-pharmaceuticals/buffetts-berkshire-acquires-5-million-shares-unitedhealth-2025-08-14/.

18. Josh Nathan-Kazis, "UnitedHealth Stock Jumps. It Cleared a Low—but Important—Hurdle," *Barron's*, September 9, 2025, accessed October 5, 2025, https://www.barrons.com/articles/united-health-care-unh-stock-price-a892bdab.

19. "Why UnitedHealth Group (UNH) Outpaced the Stock Market Today," *Yahoo Finance*, September 8, 2025, accessed October 5, 2025, https://finance.yahoo.
com/news/why-unitedhealth-group-unh-outpaced-233308149.html.

20. "UnitedHealth Group Stock Forecast," *StockAnalysis*, accessed October 5, 2025, https://stockanalysis.com/stocks/unh/forecast/.

21. "UnitedHealth Is Dropping a Million Seniors from Medicare Advantage as It Aims to Restore Its 'Swagger,'" *Morningstar/MarketWatch*, November 19, 2025, accessed January 16, 2026, https://www.morningstar.com/news/
marketwatch/20251119203/unitedhealth-is-dropping-a-million-seniors-from-medicare-advantage-as-it-aims-to-restore-its-swagger.

22. Steven Burnett, "US Insurance Industry Statistics 2025: Facts, Figures, and Emerging Trends," *CoinLaw*, June 16, 2025, accessed October 5, 2025, https://
coinlaw.io/us-insurance-industry-statistics/.

23. Wendell Potter, "UnitedHealth Group's Fight for Survival," *HEALTH CARE Un-covered* (Substack), May 21, 2025, accessed October 5, 2025, https://healthcareuncovered.substack.com/p/unitedhealth-groups-fight-for-survival.

24. Jared Ortaliza et al., "How Will the 2025 Budget Reconciliation Affect the ACA, Medicaid, and the Uninsured Rate?," KFF, June 18, 2025, accessed October 5, 2025, https://www.kff.org/affordable-care-act/how-will-the-2025-budget-reconciliation-affect-the-aca-medicaid-and-the-uninsured-rate/.

25. Jessica Hall, "Medicare Will Test Using AI to Help Decide Whether Patients Receive Coverage," *MarketWatch*, August 8, 2025, accessed October 4, 2025, https://www.marketwatch.com/story/medicare-will-test-using-ai-to-help-decide-whether-patients-receive-coverage-37a47251.

26. Reed Abelson and Teddy Rosenbluth, "Medicare Will Require Prior Approval for Certain Procedures," *The New York Times*, August 28, 2025, accessed October 5, 2025, https://www.nytimes.com/2025/08/28/health/medicare-prior-approval-health-care.html.

27. Colin Campbell, "NC Lawmakers Take Aim at Insurance Companies' 'Prior Authorization' System," *WUNC*, March 18, 2025, accessed October 5, 2025, https://www.wunc.org/politics/2025-03-18/nc-legislature-insurance-companies-prior-authorization-system.

28. Wendell Potter, *Deadly Spin: An Insurance Company Insider Speaks Out on How Corporate PR Is Killing Health Care and Deceiving Americans* (New York: Bloomsbury Press, 2010), 18.

29. Potter, *Deadly Spin,* 207.

30. Spencer Carnes, "How Medicare Advantage Is Hurting Workers," *Common Dreams*, July 3, 2025, accessed October 5, 2025, https://www.commondreams.org/opinion/medicare-advantage-scam-2672557766.

31. Christopher Weaver et al., "Insurers Pocketed $50 Billion from Medicare for Diseases No Doctor Treated," *The Wall Street Journal*, July 8, 2024, accessed October 5, 2025, https://www.wsj.com/health/healthcare/medicare-health-insurance-diagnosis-payments-b4d99a5d.

32. Reed Abelson and Margot Sanger-Katz, "'The Cash Monster Was Insatiable': How Insurers Exploited Medicare for Billions," *The New York Times*, October 8, 2022, accessed October 5, 2025, https://www.nytimes.com/2022/10/08/upshot/medicare-advantage-fraud-allegations.html.

33. Fred Schulte and Holly K. Hacker, "Hidden Audits Reveal Millions in Overcharges by Medicare Advantage Plans," NPR, November 21, 2022, accessed October 5, 2025, https://www.npr.org/sections/health-shots/2022/11/21/1137500875/audit-medicare-advantage-overcharged-medicare.

34. Ibid.

35. Wendell Potter, "Here Is the Truth: Medicare Advantage Is Neither Medicare Nor an Advantage," *Common Dreams*, January 14, 2023, accessed October 16, 2025, https://www.commondreams.org/opinion/is-medicare-advantage-a-scam.

36. Caroline Catherman, "Medicare Advantage May Cost the Government $84B More Than Traditional in 2025," *Healthcare Brew*, March 18, 2025, accessed October 5, 2025, https://www.healthcare-brew.com/stories/2025/03/18/medicare-advantage-cost-government-84-billion-2025.

37. "Why Healthcare Price Transparency Still Matters for Employers," NewCity Insurance, May 26, 2025, accessed October 5, 2025, https://newcityinsurance.com/why-healthcare-price-transparency-still-matters-for-employers/.

38. Wendell Potter, "How Insurers Obscure Healthcare Costs," *HEALTH CARE Un-covered*, accessed October 5, 2025, https://www.uncovered.health/features/how-insurers-obscure-healthcare-costs/.

39. Elisabeth Rosenthal, "GoFundMe Has Become a Health Care Utility," *KFF Health News*, February 12, 2024, accessed October 5, 2025, https://kffhealthnews.org/news/article/gofundme-health-care-funding-hospitals-surprise-bills/.

Chapter 9

1. *A Bug's Life* – "*Then They ALL Might Stand Up to Us,*" YouTube video,:45-1:00, July 17, 2010, https://www.youtube.com/watch?v=VLbWnJGlyMU. (YouTube).

2. *A Bug's Life* – "*Flik stands up to Hopper,*" YouTube video, 2:05–2:22, accessed October 2, 2025. https://www.youtube.com/watch?v=g0UabjeVnU8.

3. Collin Rugg (@CollinRugg), "AOC Fights Back Tears, Calls the Passing of Trump's Bill 'One of the Saddest Days in Modern American History'," X, July 3, 2025, https://x.com/CollinRugg/status/1940872198690164908.

4. DocGlauc (@docglauc), *Instagram reel*, August 15, 2025, https://www.instagram.com/reel/DNYvmYdqphZ/.

5. Michael J. Alkire, "Unnecessary Insurance Claim Denials Compromise Patient Care and Provider Bottom Lines," *STAT*, May 1, 2024, https://www.statnews.com/2024/05/01/insurance-claim-denials-compromise-patient-care-provider-bottom-lines/.

6. Sara R. Collins, Lauren A. Haynes, and Relebohile Masitha, "The State of U.S. Health Insurance in 2022: Findings from the Commonwealth Fund Biennial Health Insurance Survey" Commonwealth Fund, Sept. 29, 2022, https://www

.commonwealthfund.org/publications/issue-briefs/2022/sep/state-us-health-insurance-2022-biennial-survey.

7. Claremont Insurance Services, "KFF 2024 Employer Health Benefits Survey," October 28, 2024, https://www.claremontcompanies.com/kff-2024-employer-health-benefits-survey/.

8. Centers for Medicare & Medicaid Services, *Health Insurance Exchanges 2025 Open Enrollment Report* (2024), https://www.cms.gov/files/document/health-insurance-exchanges-2025-open-enrollment-report.pdf.

9. Kaiser Family Foundation (KFF), "About Half of Adults with ACA Market-place Coverage Are Small-Business Owners, Employees, or Self-Employed," KFF, May 2024, https://www.kff.org/affordable-care-act/about-half-of-adults-with-aca-marketplace-coverage-are-small-business-owners-employees-or-self-employed/.

10. KFF, *"About Half of Adults with ACA Marketplace Coverage"* (May 2024).

11. U.S. Census Bureau, "2024 Presidential Election Voting and Registration Tables," *Newsroom Press Release*, April 30, 2025, https://www.census.gov/newsroom/press-releases/2025/2024-presidential-election-voting-registration-tables.html.

12. American Cancer Society, "Cancer Facts & Figures 2025" (Atlanta: American Cancer Society, 2025), https://www.cancer.org/content/dam/cancer-org/research/cancer-facts-and-statistics/annual-cancer-facts-and-figures/2025/2025-cancer-facts-and-figures-acs.pdf.

13. Stephen Gutowski, "NRA Membership Fell to 3.8 Million in 2023," *The Reload*, July 12, 2024, https://thereload.com/nra-membership-fell-to-3-8-million-in-2023/.

14. Mike Johnson, "Speaker Johnson: The President is waiting with his pen. And the American people are waiting for relief," press release, May 22, 2025, https://mikejohnson.house.gov/news/documentsingle.aspx?DocumentID=1600.

15. UnitedHealth Group, *Investor Conference 2024 Book*, 8 (2024), https://www.unitedhealthgroup.com/content/dam/UHG/PDF/investors/2024/ic24/Investor-Conference-2024-Book.pdf.

16. Alexis Kayser, "Hospitals Are Reporting More Insurance Denials. Is AI Driving Them?" *Newsweek*, November 14, 2024, https://www.newsweek.com/hospitals-are-reporting-more-insurance-denials-ai-driving-them-1977706.

17. Elizabeth Napolitano, "UnitedHealth uses faulty AI to deny elderly patients medically necessary coverage, lawsuit claims," *CBS News*, November 20, 2023, https://www.cbsnews.com/news/unitedhealth-lawsuit-ai-deny-claims-medicare-advantage-health-insurance-denials/.

18. Patrick Rucker, Maya Miller, and David Armstrong, "How Cigna Saves Millions by Having Its Doctors Reject Claims Without Reading Them," ProPublica, March 25, 2023, https://www.propublica.org/article/cigna-pxdx-medical-health-insurance-rejection-claims.

19. Rucker, Miller, and Armstrong, "How Cigna Saves Millions by Having Its Doctors Reject Claims Without Reading Them."

20. Bruce Japsen, "Health Insurers Vow to Simplify and Reduce Pre-Approval Process," *Forbes*, June 23, 2025, https://www.forbes.com/sites/brucejapsen/2025/06/23/health-insurers-vow-to-simplify-and-reduce-pre-approval-process/.

21. "Navigating the American Healthcare System: South Park: The End of Obesity," YouTube video, 1:19–1:31 May 27, 2024, https://www.youtube.com/watch?v=VAfy26xs6e0.

22. Gary Claxton, Cynthia Cox, Anthony Damico, Larry Levitt, and Karen Pollitz, "Pre-Existing Condition Prevalence for Individuals and Families," KFF, October 4, 2019, https://www.kff.org/affordable-care-act/pre-existing-condition-prevalence-for-individuals-and-families/.

23. Claxton, Cox, Damico, Levitt, and Pollitz, "Pre-Existing Condition Prevalence for Individuals and Families."

24. American Cancer Society Cancer Action Network (ACS CAN), "Survivor Views: Majority of Cancer Patients & Survivors Have or Expect to Have Medical Debt," May 9, 2024, https://www.fightcancer.org/policy-resources/survivor-views-majority-cancer-patients-survivors-have-or-expect-have-medical-debt.

25. Jen Smith, "Prior Authorization Linked to Cancer Progression and Death," *Cancer Therapy Advisor*, November 29, 2022, https://www.cancertherapyadvisor.com/news/prior-authorization-linked-cancer-progression-death/.

26. Smith, "Prior Authorization Linked to Cancer Progression and Death."

27. American Cancer Society Cancer Action Network (ACS CAN), "Survey: Cancer Patients and Survivors Alter or Delay Care Due to Insurance Barriers," December 5, 2019, https://www.fightcancer.org/releases/survey-cancer-patients-and-survivors-alter-or-delay-care-due-insurance-barriers.

28. ACS CAN, "Survivor Views: Majority of Cancer Patients & Survivors Have or Expect to Have Medical Debt."

29. "42% of cancer patients spent entire life savings in 2 years after diagnosis, study finds" *Advisory*, November 1, 2018, updated September 15, 2023. https://www.advisory.com/daily-briefing/2018/11/01/financial-toxicity.

30. Nora Kenworthy and Mark Igra, "Medical Crowdfunding and Disparities in Health Care Access in the United States, 2016–2020," *American Journal of Public Health* 112, no. 3 (March 2022): 491–498, https://doi.org/10.2105/AJPH.2021.306617.

31. Richard Westlund, "Study Points to Significant Disparities in Federal Cancer Research Funding," *University of Miami News*, June 8, 2023, https://news.med.miami.edu/study-points-to-significant-disparities-in-federal-cancer-research-funding/.

32. Jeremy Elias, "Where Have All the Educated Consumers Gone?," *Tablet*, November 2, 2021, https://www.tabletmag.com/sections/community/articles/educated-consumers-syms.

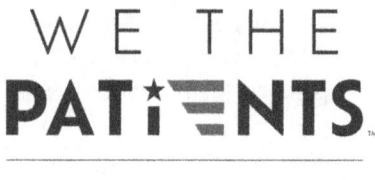

WETHEPATIENTS.ORG

For more information about the movement, visit WeThePatients.org.

Index